AROMATHERAPY A-Z

CONNIE AND ALAN HIGLEY
AND
PAT LEATHAM

Hay House, Inc.
Carlsbad, California • Sydney, Australia
Canada • Hong Kong • United Kingdom

Published and distributed in the United States by:

Hay House, Inc., P.O. Box 5100, Carlsbad, CA 92018-5100 • (800) 654-5126 • (800) 650-5115 (fax)

Designed by: Tom Morgan, Blue Design

Library of Congress Cataloging-in-Publication Data

Higley, Connie.
   Aromatherapy a-z / Connie Higley, and Alan Higley, and Pat Leatham.
p. cm.
ISBN 1-56170-489-X (hbk.) • ISBN: 1-56170-796-1 (tradepaper)
   1. Aromatherapy—Encyclopedias.   I. Higley, Alan.   II. Leatham, Pat.   III. Title.
   RM666.A68H54   1998
   615'.321—dc21

                        97-53183
                        CIP

ISBN 1-56170-796-1

05 04 03 02   6 5 4 3
1st printing, June 1998
3rd printing, August 2002

Printed in China through Palace Press International

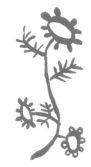

DISCLAIMER

The information contained in this document was gathered and put together for the personal use of the compilers. The compilers of this document have no expertise in the area of nutrition, but are merely users of essential oils and other natural health-care products. The information for this document was obtained from lectures, books, newsletters about essential oils, personal experiences, and from the successful experiences of others. Although every effort has been made to ensure accuracy, it is not guaranteed to be 100 percent accurate. It was compiled in this way to enable the compilers easy access to the information that they have gathered. It is not provided in order to diagnose, prescribe, or treat any disease, illness, or injured condition of the body. Furthermore, neither the compilers of this document nor any maker or distributor of essential oils assumes responsibility for such use. Each person will have to use his or her own intuition in deciding which oil to use for a particular problem. Each person is different; an oil that works for one individual may not work for another. Anyone suffering from any disease, illness, or injury should consult a physician.

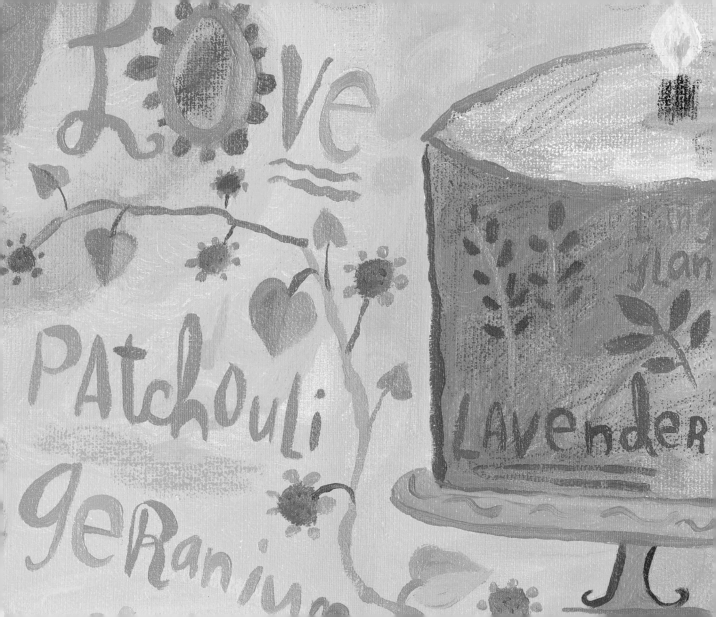

Contents

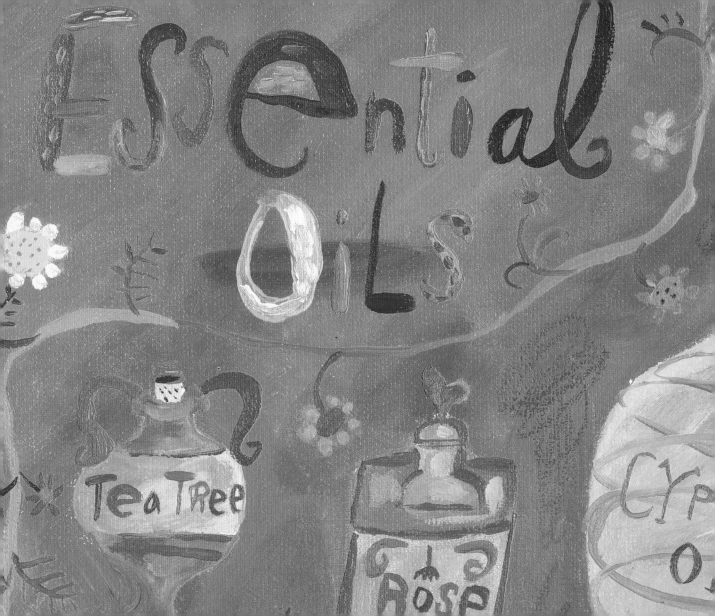

Basic Facts about Essential Oils

HOW LONG HAVE ESSENTIAL OILS BEEN AROUND?

Essential oils were humankind's first medicine. From Egyptian hieroglyphics and Chinese manuscripts, we know that priests and physicians have been using essential oils for thousands of years. In Egypt, essential oils were used in the embalming process, and well-preserved oils were found in alabaster jars in King Tut's tomb. Egyptian temples were dedicated to the production and blending of the oils, and recipes were recorded on the walls in hieroglyphics. There is even a sacred room in the temple of Isis on the island of Philae where a ritual called "Cleansing the Flesh and Blood of Evil Deities" was practiced. This form of emotional clearing required three days of cleansing, using particular essential oils and oil baths.

There are 188 references to essential oils in the Bible. Oils such as frankincense, myrrh, rosemary, hyssop, and spikenard were used for anointing and healing the sick. In Exodus, the Lord gave the following recipe to Moses for "an holy anointing oil":
Myrrh ("five hundred shekels"—approximately 1 gallon)
Sweet Cinnamon ("two hundred and fifty shekels"— approximately 1/2 gallon)
Sweet Calamus ("two hundred and fifty shekels")
Cassia ("five hundred shekels")
Olive Oil ("an hin"—approximately 1/3 gallon)

The three wise men presented the Christ child with essential oils of frankincense and myrrh. There are also accounts in the New Testament of the Bible where Jesus was anointed with spikenard oil: "And being in Bethany in the house of Simon the leper, as he sat at meat, there came a woman having an alabaster box of ointment of spikenard very precious; and she brake the box, and poured [it] on his head" (Mark 14:3). "Then took Mary a pound of ointment of spikenard, very costly, and anointed the feet of Jesus, and wiped his feet with her hair: and the house was filled with the odour of the ointment" (John 12:3).

WHAT ARE PURE (GRADE A) ESSENTIAL OILS?

Essential oils are the volatile liquids that are distilled from plants (including their respective parts such as seeds, bark, leaves, stems, roots, flowers, fruit, etc.). One of the factors that determines the purity of an oil is its chemical constituents. These constituents can be affected by a vast number of variables, including the part(s) of the plant from which the oil was produced, soil condition, fertilizer (organic or chemical), geographical region, climate, altitude, harvest season and methods, and distillation process. For example, common thyme, or thyme vulgaris, produces several different chemotypes (biochemical specifics or simple species), depending on the conditions of its growth, climate, and altitude. One will produce high levels of thymol, depending on the time of year it is distilled. If distilled during midsummer or late fall, it can contain higher levels of carvacrol, which can cause the oil to be more caustic or irritating to the skin. Low pressure and low temperature are also keys to maintaining the purity, ultimate fragrance, and therapeutic value of the oil.

As we begin to understand the power of essential oils in the realm of personal, holistic health care, we comprehend the absolute necessity for obtaining the purest essential oils possible. Chemists have yet to successfully recreate essential oils in the laboratory.

The information in this book is based upon the use of pure, grade-A essential oils. Those who are beginning their journey into the realm of aromatherapy and essential oils must actively seek for the purest quality oils available. Anything less than pure may not produce the desired results.

WHAT BENEFITS DO PURE ESSENTIAL OILS PROVIDE?

1. Essential oils are the regenerating, oxygenating, and immune defense properties of plants.
2. Essential oils are so small in molecular size that they can quickly penetrate the tissues of the skin.
3. Essential oils are lipid soluble and are capable of penetrating cell walls, even if they have hardened because of an oxygen deficiency. In fact, essential oils can affect every cell of the body within 20 minutes and are then metabolized like other nutrients.
4. Essential oils contain oxygen molecules that help to transport nutrients to the starving human cells. Because a nutritional deficiency is an oxygen deficiency, disease begins when the cells lack the oxygen for proper nutrient assimilation. By providing the needed oxygen, essential oils also work to help stimulate the immune mechanisms of the body.

5. Essential oils are very powerful antioxidants. Antioxidants create an unfriendly environment for free radicals. They prevent all mutations, work as free radical scavengers, prevent fungus, and prevent oxidation in the cells.

6. Essential oils can be antibacterial, anticancerous, antifungal, anti-infectious, antimicrobial, antitumoral, antiparasitic, antiviral, and antiseptic. Some essential oils have been shown to destroy all tested bacteria and viruses while simultaneously restoring balance to the body.

7. Essential oils may detoxify the cells and blood in the body.

8. Essential oils containing sesquiterpenes have the ability to pass the blood-brain barrier, enabling them to be effective in the treatment of Alzheimer's disease, Lou Gehrig's disease, Parkinson's disease, and multiple sclerosis.

9. Essential oils are aromatic. When diffused, they provide air purification by:
   a. Removing metallic particles and toxins from the air;
   b. Increasing atmospheric oxygen;
   c. Increasing ozone and negative ions in the area, which inhibits bacterial growth;
   d. Destroying odors from mold, cigarettes, and animals; and
   e. Filling the air with a fresh, aromatic scent.

10. Essential oils help promote emotional, physical, and spiritual healing.

11. Essential oils have a bioelectrical frequency that is several times greater than the frequency of herbs, food, and even the human body. Clinical research has shown that essential oils have the potential to quickly raise the frequency of the human body, restoring it to its normal, healthy level.

WHAT IS FREQUENCY, AND HOW DOES IT PERTAIN TO PURE ESSENTIAL OILS?

Frequency is a measurable rate of electrical energy that is constant between any two points. Everything has an electrical frequency. As measured in megahertz (MHZ), grade-A essential oils range from 52–320 MHZ.

Bruce Tainio of Tainio Technology in Cheny, Washington, developed new equipment to measure the bio-frequency of humans and foods. Bruce Tainio and Dr. D. Gary Young, a North American expert in the field of aromatherapy, used this bio-frequency monitor to determine the relationship between frequency and disease. Some of the results of their studies are as follows.

HUMANS

Human brain	72–90 MHZ
Human body (daytime)	62–68 MHZ
Cold symptoms	58 MHZ
Flu symptoms	57 MHZ
Candida	55 MHZ
Epstein Barr	52 MHZ
Cancer	42 MHZ
Death begins	25 MHZ

FOODS

Processed/canned food	0 MHZ
Fresh produce	up to 15 MHZ
Dry herbs	12–22 MHZ
Fresh herbs	20–27 MHZ
Essential oils	52–320 MHZ

Another part of these same studies measured the frequency fluctuations within the human body as different substances were introduced. In one case, the frequency of each of two different individuals—the first a 26-year-old male and the second a 24-year-old male—was measured at 66 MHZ for both. The first individual held a cup of coffee (without drinking any), and his frequency dropped to 58 MHZ in 3 seconds. He then removed the coffee and inhaled an aroma of essential oils. Within 21 seconds, his frequency had returned to 66 MHZ. The second individual took a sip of coffee, and his frequency dropped to 52 MHZ in the same 3 seconds. However, no essential oils were used during the recovery time, and it took three days for his frequency to return to the initial 66 MHZ.

Another interesting result of these studies was the influence that thoughts have on our frequency as well. Negative thoughts lowered the measured frequency by 12 MHZ, and positive thoughts raised the measured frequency by 10 MHZ. It was also found that prayer and meditation increased the measured frequency levels by 15 MHZ.

WHAT EFFECT DO PURE ESSENTIAL OILS HAVE ON THE BRAIN?

The blood-brain barrier is the barrier membrane between the circulating blood and the brain that prevents certain damaging substances from reaching brain tissue and cerebrospinal fluid. The American Medical Association (AMA) determined that if it could find an agent that would pass the blood-brain barrier, it would be able to cure Alzheimer's disease, Lou Gehrig's disease, multiple sclerosis, and Parkinson's disease. In June 1994, it was documented by the Medical University of Berlin, Germany; and Vienna, Austria, that sesquiterpenes have the ability to go beyond the blood-brain barrier.

High levels of sesquiterpenes, found in the essential oils of frankincense and sandalwood, help increase the amount of oxygen in the limbic system of the brain, particularly around the pineal and pituitary glands. This leads to an increase in secretions of antibodies, endorphins, and neurotransmitters.

Also present in the limbic system of the brain is a gland called the amygdala. In 1989, it was discovered that the amygdala plays a major role in storing and releasing emotional trauma. The only way to stimulate this gland is with fragrance or the sense of smell. Therefore, with aromatherapy and essential oils, we now have an effective means to help with the release of emotional trauma.

WHAT ENABLES PURE ESSENTIAL OILS TO PROVIDE SUCH INCREDIBLE BENEFITS?

Essential oils are chemically heterogeneous, meaning they are very diverse in their effects and can perform several different functions. Synthetic chemicals are completely opposite in that they have basically one action. This gives essential oils a paradoxical nature that can be difficult to understand. However, they can be compared with another paradoxical group— human beings. For example, a man can play many roles: father, husband, friend, co-worker, accountant, school teacher, church volunteer, scout master, minister. etc., and so it is with essential oils. Lavender can be used for burns, insect bites, headaches, PMS, insomnia, stress and so forth.

The heterogeneous benefits of an oil depend greatly on its chemical constituents—not only on the existence of specific constituents, but also their amounts in proportion to the other constituents that are present in the same oil. Some individual oils may have anywhere from 200 to 800 different chemical constituents. However, of the possible 800 different constituents, only about 200 of those have so far been identified. Although not everything is known about all the different constituents, most of them can be grouped into a few distinct families, each with some dominant characteristics.

Application of Essential Oils

DIFFUSE

The easiest and simplest way of putting the oils into the air for inhalation is to use an aromatic diffuser. Diffusers that use a heat source (such as a lightbulb ring) can alter the chemical makeup of the oil and its therapeutic qualities. A cold air diffuser uses room-temperature air to blow the oil up against a nebulizer. This breaks the oils up into a micro-fine mist that is then dispersed into the air, covering thousands of square feet in seconds. The oils, with their oxygenating molecules, will then remain suspended for several hours to freshen and improve the quality of the air. The antiviral, antibacterial, and antiseptic properties of the oils, as well as negative ions, kill bacteria and help to reduce fungus and mold. Essential oils, when diffused, have been found to reduce the amount of airborne chemicals and metallics, as well as help to create greater physical, spiritual, and emotional harmony. It is usually best to diffuse an oil for only 15 to 30 minutes at a time and gradually increase these periods as you become accustomed to it.

DIRECT APPLICATION

Essential oils can be applied directly on the area of concern using one to six drops. More oil is not necessarily better; one to three drops is usually adequate. Some oils may need to be diluted with a pure vegetable oil.

BODY MASSAGE

If massaging a large area of the body, always dilute the oils by 15 to 30 percent with a pure vegetable oil.

FEET MASSAGE

Your feet are the second fastest area of your body to absorb oils because of the large pores. Three to six drops per foot are adequate to experience a feeling of peace, relaxation, or energy.

VITA FLEX THERAPY

One to three drops of oil may be applied to the Vita Flex points (nerve ending points) on the foot (refer to the following Vita Flex Feet Chart). The oils can then be worked into the foot by using a technique of curl, press, and release; start with the tips of the fingers, curl over onto the fingernails—increasing pressure during the curl—then release. This technique can bring some tremendous relief to tired, aching feet, as well as send the oil along the nerve to affect the organ at the other end.

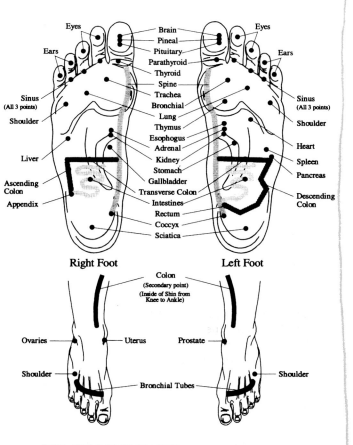

Right Foot **Left Foot**

Eyes — Brain — Pineal — Pituitary — Parathyroid — Thyroid — Spine — Trachea — Bronchial — Lung — Thymus — Esophogus — Adrenal — Kidney — Stomach — Gallbladder — Transverse Colon — Intestines — Rectum — Coccyx — Sciatica — Eyes

Ears — Ears

Sinus (All 3 points) — Sinus (All 3 points)

Shoulder — Shoulder

Liver — Heart

Ascending Colon — Spleen

Appendix — Pancreas

Descending Colon

Colon (Secondary point) (Inside of Shin from Knee to Ankle)

Ovaries — Uterus — Prostate

Shoulder — Shoulder

Bronchial Tubes

VITA FLEX FEET CHART

AURICULAR THERAPY

Applying essential oils to the rim of the ear is known as *auricular therapy*. As with the feet, many internal organs have nerve endings in the ears. Try using different oils on the ears to help with emotional clearing.

RAINDROP THERAPY

This technique of dropping essential oils on the spine helps bring the body into balance, aligns the energy centers of the body, and releases them if blocked. The oils used in this therapy help to kill any viruses and bacteria that may be hibernating along the spine and will continue to work in the body for about 5 to 7 days after the treatment. The following oils are used: thyme, oregano, cypress, birch, basil, peppermint, and marjoram. Pure vegetable oil is used to help reduce the burning sensation produced by some of these oils. A moist, hot towel can also be applied along the length of the spine to help force the oils deeper into the skin. Placing a dry towel on top of the wet towel helps to contain the moist heat.

BATHS

Add three to six drops of oil to 1/2 oz. of a bath and shower gel base and add to the water while the tub is filling. The number of drops can be increased as you become accustomed to the oils.

PERFUME OR COLOGNE

Wearing the oils as a perfume or cologne can provide not only a beautiful fragrance but also some wonderful emotional and physical support.

Guide for Using Essential Oils

HOW TO USE THE GUIDE

1. *Aromatic* means diffuse, breathe, or inhale.
2. An asterisk (*) means that the oil has been proven in the clinics in Europe (France).
3. *Neat* means to apply the oil without diluting it with a pure vegetable oil.
4. If essential oils get in your eyes by accident or they burn a little, do not try to remove the oils with water. This will only drive them deeper into the tissue. It is best to dilute the essential oils with a pure vegetable oil.
5. Essential oils should only be applied topically. The FDA has not approved essential oils for internal use.
6. Using citrus oils such as lemon, orange, grapefruit, mandarin, bergamot, angelica, etc. during exposure to direct sunlight may cause a rash or pigmentation. It is best to dilute the oil first with a pure vegetable oil, then apply a small amount to determine how the skin responds.
7. Extreme caution should be used with oils such as clary sage, sage, and fennel during pregnancy. These oils contain active constituents with hormonelike activity and could possibly cause an abortion, though there are no recorded cases in humans.
8. Particular care should be taken when using cinnamon, lemongrass, oregano, and thyme because these are some of the strongest and most caustic oils. It is best to dilute them with a pure vegetable oil.
9. Essential oils are not listed in a specific order (an attempt was made to list them alphabetically), so you will have to be intuitive on which one to use. It is not necessary to use all of the oils listed. Try one oil at a time. If you do not see a change soon, try a different one. What one person needs may be different from another person. (*Hint*: Use Kinesiology to test yourself on the oils that are right for you.)
10. In this guide, several homemade blends are suggested. However, it is done with great hesitancy. Some of the blends listed come from individuals who may not be experts in the field of essential oils and aromatherapy.

Rather than mix the oils together, it is better to layer the oils; that is, apply one oil, rub it in, and then apply another oil. If dilution is necessary, a pure vegetable oil can be applied on top.

11. When someone is out of balance, try the following:
    a. Place one drop each of hyssop, spruce, lavender, spikenard, and geranium in one hand, then rub the palms of both hands together in a clockwise motion.
    b. Place one hand over the thymus (heart chakra) and the other hand over the navel.
    c. Take three deep breaths and switch hands, then take three more deep breaths.

12. Less is often better; use one to three drops of oil and no more than six drops at a time. Stir and rub on in a clockwise direction.

13. When applying oils to infants and small children, dilute with a pure vegetable oil. Use one to three drops of essential oil to 1 tablespoon (Tbl.) of vegetable oil for infants, and one to three drops of essential oil to 1 teaspoon (tsp.) vegetable oil for children two to five years old.

14. The body absorbs oils the fastest through inhalation (breathing) and second fastest through application to the feet or ears.

Testing on the thyroid, heart, and pancreas showed that the oils reached these organs in three seconds. Layering the oils can increase the rate of absorption.

15. When an oil causes discomfort, it is because it is pulling toxins, heavy metals, chemicals, poisons, parasites, and mucus from the system. Either stop applying the oils for a short time, to make sure your body isn't eliminating (detoxifying) too fast, or dilute the oils until the body catches up with the releasing. These toxins go back into the system if they cannot be released.

16. When the cell wall thickens, oxygen cannot get in. The life expectancy of the cell is 120 days (4 months). Cells divide, making two duplicate cells. If the cell is diseased, two new diseased cells will be made. When we stop the mutation of the cells (create healthy cells), we stop the disease. Essential oils have the ability to penetrate and carry nutrients through the cell wall to the nucleus and improve the health of the cell.

17. Each oil has a frequency, and each of our organs and body parts has a frequency. The frequency of an oil is attracted by a like frequency within the body. Lower oil frequencies become a sponge for negative energy. The frequency is what stays in the body to maintain the longer-lasting effects of the oil.

Low frequencies can make **physical** changes in the body.
Middle frequencies can make **emotional** changes in the body.
High frequencies can make **spiritual** changes in the body.

a.   Average frequency of the human body during the daytime is between 62 and 68 MHZ.

   1) Bone frequency is 38 to 43 MHZ.

   2) Frequencies from the neck down vary between 62 and 68 MHZ.

b.   Spiritual frequencies range from 92 to 360 MHZ.

18. *Use extreme caution when diffusing cinnamon bark* because it may burn the nostrils if you put your nose directly next to the nebulizer of the diffuser.

19. When traveling by air, you should always have your oils hand-checked. X-ray machines may interfere with the frequency of the oils.

20. Keep oils away from light and heat, although they seem to do fine in temperatures up to 90 degrees. If stored properly, they can maintain their maximum potency for many years.

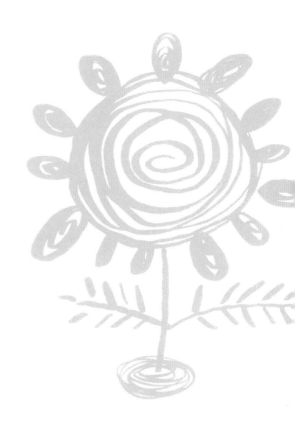

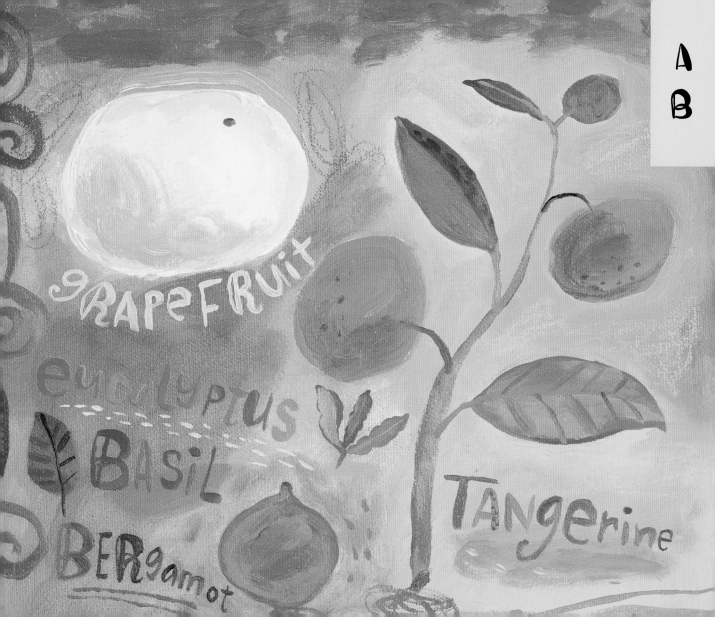

GRAPEFRUIT

eucalyptus

BASIL

BERgamot

TANGERINE

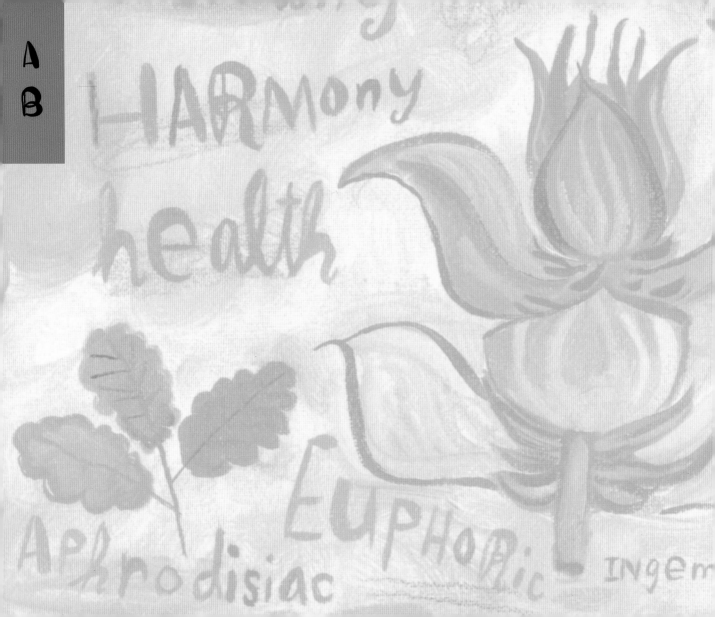

CONDITIONS AND TREATMENTS

ABSCESS

Thyme*; hot compress of bergamot, chamomile, lavender, or melaleuca.

MOUTH

Lavender*

ABSENTMINDED

Basil

ABUNDANCE

Bergamot

ATTRACTS

Cinnamon bark

MONEY

Ginger, patchouly

ABUSE

Geranium, sandalwood, ylang-ylang. Apply one drop of the oils desired on each chakra to allow blocked emotions to come out.

BY FATHER

Lavender

BY MOTHER

Geranium, lavender

SEXUAL

Sage

ACHES

Birch, bergamot, cedarwood, chamomile, eucalyptus, fir, helichrysum and spruce (for pain), juniper, lavender, lemon, marjoram*

ACID

(SEE pH BALANCE)

Putting 1 or 2 drops of peppermint in drinking water, on stomach, and/or on feet may help.

ACNE

Bergamot, cedarwood, chamomile, clary sage, eucalyptus, juniper*, lavender*, lemon, marjoram, melaleuca, patchouly, rosemary, rosewood*, sage, thyme. Apply one of these oils directly on location.

ADDICTIONS

Bergamot (helps with overindulgences such as alcohol, coffee, tea, tobacco)

COFFEE/TOBACCO

Bergamot. Apply to stomach, abdomen, liver area, and bottoms of feet.

DRUGS

Basil, bergamot, birch, chamomile (Roman), eucalyptus, fennel, grapefruit (withdrawal), lavender, marjoram, nutmeg, orange, sandalwood.

WITHDRAWAL

Grapefruit, lavender, marjoram, nutmeg, orange, sandalwood. Apply to temples and diffuse.

ADRENAL CORTEX

Nutmeg has adrenal cortex properties. It may also help support and increase energy.

STIMULATE

Basil*, sage*

STRENGTHEN

Spruce (black), peppermint

AGENT ORANGE

Bathe in Epsom salts and 4 oz. of food-grade peroxide.

AGING

(SEE WRINKLES)

Frankincense, sandalwood

AGITATION

Bergamot, cedarwood, clary sage, frankincense, geranium, juniper, lavender, marjoram, myrrh, rose, rosewood, sandalwood, ylang-ylang

AIDS

Apply nutmeg* to thymus and bottoms of feet.

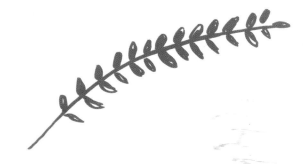

AIR POLLUTION

Cypress, eucalyptus, fir (fights airborne germs and bacteria), grapefruit, lavender, lemon, rosemary

DISINFECTANT

Lemon*

ALCOHOL

(SEE ADDICTIONS)

Fennel, juniper, and rosemary

ALERTNESS

Basil, peppermint, rosemary; apply to temples and bottoms of feet.

ALKALINE

(SEE pH BALANCE)

The body can only heal itself in an alkaline state.

ALLERGIES

Eucalyptus, lavender*, patchouly*, peppermint, raven; apply to sinuses, bottoms of feet, and diffuse.
Apply 1 drop of peppermint on the base of the neck twice daily. Tap the thymus (located just below the notch in the neck) with pointer and index fingers (energy fingers). Diffuse peppermint. The use of peppermint may result in no more allergy shots.

HAY FEVER *(SEE HAY FEVER)*

RASHES, SKIN SENSITIVITY

Apply 3 drops lavender, 6 drops chamomile (Roman), 2 drops myrrh, and 1 drop peppermint on location.

ALZHEIMER'S DISEASE

Cypress; apply to temples, bottoms of feet, and diffuse.

ANALGESIC

Birch, eucalyptus, helichrysum, lavender, lemongrass, marjoram, melaleuca, oregano, peppermint, rosemary

ANEMIA

Lavender, lemon*; apply to stomach and bottoms of feet.

ANESTHESIA

Helichrysum

ANEURYSM

Blend: Combine 5 drops frankincense, 1 drop helichrysum, and 1 drop cypress. Diffuse.

ANGER

Bergamot, cedarwood, chamomile (Roman and blue), frankincense, lavender, lemon, mandarin, marjoram, melissa, myrrh

(soothes), myrtle, orange, petitgrain, rose, sandalwood, ylang-ylang

CALMS

Spruce

CLEANSING AFTER ARGUMENT AND PHYSICAL FIGHTING

Eucalyptus

DISPELS

Ylang-ylang

COMMUNICATION WITHOUT ANGER

Chamomile

LESSENS

Myrrh

OVERCOMES

Bergamot, cedarwood*, chamomile

RELEASES LOCKED-UP ANGER AND FRUSTRATION

Sandalwood
Blend: Combine 4 drops lavender, 3 drops geranium, 3 drops rosewood, 3 drops rosemary, 2 drops tangerine, 1 drop spearmint, 2 drops tansy, 2 drops blue chamomile, and 1 oz. pure vegetable oil. Apply to back of neck, wrist, and heart.

ANGINA

Ginger*, orange* (for false angina); apply to heart.

ANOREXIA

Grapefruit, tarragon; apply to stomach and bottoms of feet. It may also help to diffuse.

ANTHRAX

(Animal disease found in cows and sheep; can be transmitted to humans.) Thyme*

ANTI-AGING

Rosewood

ANTIBACTERIAL

Basil*, bergamot, cassia, cedarwood, chamomile, citronella, citrus oils, cinnamon*, clary sage, clove*, cypress*, eucalyptus, fir*, geranium, grapefruit, juniper*, lavender, lemon, nutmeg*

(intestinal), marjoram, melaleuca*, mountain savory, neroli, oregano*, palmarosa, petitgrain, ravensara, rosemary*, rosewood*, spearmint*, tarragon, thyme*, wild tansy

AIRBORNE

Fir

INFECTION

Nutmeg (fights)

ANTIBIOTIC

Bergamot, chamomile (Roman), cinnamon, clove, eucalyptus, hyssop, lavender, lemon, melaleuca, myrtle, nutmeg, oregano, patchouly, ravensara, thyme; apply on location, liver area, bottoms of feet, and diffuse.

ANTICANCEROUS

Clove, frankincense

ANTICATARRHAL

Cypress*, eucalyptus, fir, frankincense*, ginger, helichrysum* (discharges mucus), hyssop (opens respiratory system and discharges toxins and mucous), jasmine, pepper (black), ravensara, and rosemary; apply on lung area, feet, around nose, and diffuse.

ANTICOAGULANT

Angelica, cassia, helichrysum*, lavender, tangerine; apply on location, bottoms of feet, and diffuse.

ANTIDEPRESSANT

(SEE DEPRESSION)

Frankincense*, lavender. Apply to bottoms of feet, heart, and diffuse.

ANTIFUNGAL

Cinnamon*, clove*, juniper, lavender, lemon, lemongrass, mandarin, melaleuca*, mountain savory, oregano*, palmarosa, rosewood*, spearmint*, thyme*; apply to bottoms of feet, on location, and diffuse. Blend: Combine 2 drops myrrh and 2 drops lavender; rub on location.

ANTIHEMORRHAGING

Rose

ANTIHISTAMINE

Chamomile, lavender. Apply to sinuses, diffuse.

ANTI-INFECTIOUS

Basil*, cassia, chamomile, cinnamon*, clove, cypress*, davana, eucalyptus, hyssop, lavender*, marjoram, melaleuca, myrrh, neroli, patchouly*, petitgrain, ravensara, rose, rosemary*, rosewood*, spearmint, spruce*, tarragon, thyme*, wild tansy. Apply on location and bottoms of feet.

ANTI-INFLAMMATORY

Birch*, citronella, coriander, cypress, eucalyptus, helichrysum, hyssop (of the pulmonary), lavender*, lemongrass, melaleuca, myrrh*, patchouly, pepper (black), peppermint, petitgrain, ravensara*, spearmint, spruce*, tangerine, tarragon*. Apply on location.

ANTIMICROBIAL

Cinnamon, cypress, helichrysum, jasmine, lavender, lemongrass, myrrh, palmarosa, rosemary, rosewood, sage, thyme

ANTIMUCUS

(SEE ANTICATARRHAL)

ANTIOXIDANTS

Cinnamon bark, chamomile, frankincense, helichrysum, hyssop, melaleuca, oregano, ravensara, thyme
Tea: Gojo berry

ANTIPARASITIC

Cinnamon*, clove, fennel, ginger, hyssop, lemongrass, melaleuca, mountain savory, neroli, oregano, rosemary, rosewood, spearmint, tarragon. Apply to stomach, liver, intestines, and feet.

ANTIRHEUMATIC

Birch, eucalyptus, juniper, oregano, rosemary, thyme

ANTISEPTIC

Bergamot, black cumin, cedarwood, chamomile (Roman), cinnamon, citronella, clove, eucalyptus, fennel, fir, lavender, lemon, mandarin, marjoram, melaleuca, myrtle, nutmeg* (intestinal), orange, oregano*, patchouly*, peppermint*, ravensara*, rosemary, sage*, sandalwood*, spearmint*, thyme*, ylang-ylang. Apply on location.

ANTISEXUAL

Marjoram* helps balance sexual desires.

ANTISPASMODIC

Basil*, black cumin, chamomile (relaxes spastic muscles of the colon wall, only relaxing abnormal muscles not normal muscles), citronella, fennel, helichrysum, lavender*, mandarin, marjoram*, peppermint*, petitgrain, rosemary*, sage*, spearmint, spruce*, tarragon, ylang-ylang

ANTITUMORAL

Clove, frankincense*

ANTIVIRAL

Bergamot, cinnamon, clary sage, eucalyptus, galbanum, geranium, hyssop, juniper, lavender, lemon, cinnamon*, clove*, melaleuca*, melissa, oregano*, palmarosa, ravensara*, rosewood* sandalwood, tarragon, thyme*, wild tansy

ANXIETY

Bergamot, cedarwood, chamomile, clary sage, cypress, frankincense, geranium, hyssop, jasmine, juniper, lavender, lemon, marjoram, melissa, patchouly, rose, sandalwood, tangerine, ylang-ylang

APATHY

Frankincense, geranium, jasmine, marjoram, orange, peppermint, rose, rosemary, rosewood, sandalwood, thyme, ylang-ylang

APHRODISIAC

Cinnamon*, clary sage*, ginger, jasmine, patchouly*, rose, sandalwood*, neroli, ylang-ylang*

APPETITE (LOSS OF)

Bergamot*, ginger, nutmeg*; apply to stomach, bottoms of feet, and diffuse.

ARGUMENTATIVE

Cedarwood, chamomile (Roman), eucalyptus, frankincense, jasmine, orange, thyme, ylang-ylang

ARMS (FLABBY)

Cypress, fennel, juniper, lavender

ARTERIAL VASODILATOR

Marjoram*; apply to carotids in neck, heart, and feet.

ARTERIES (BLOCKED)

Lavender

ARTERIOSCLEROSIS

Birch, ginger, juniper, lemon, rosemary, thyme. Apply to heart and feet.

ARTHRITIS

Birch, cedarwood, chamomile, clove, cypress*, eucalyptus, fir, ginger, hyssop, lavender, marjoram*, nutmeg, peppermint, rosemary*, spruce*; apply oils on location and diffuse.
Tea: Gojo berry

OSTEOARTHRITIS

Basil, birch, eucalyptus, lavender, lemon, marjoram, thyme

PAIN

Birch

RHEUMATOID (SEE RHEUMATISM)

ASTHMA
(SEE RESPIRATORY SYSTEM)

Cypress, eucalyptus*, fir, frankincense* (on crown), hyssop, lavender, lemon*, marjoram*, myrrh, myrtle, oregano*, peppermint, ravensara*, rose, rosemary, sage*, thyme*; apply topically over lungs and throat, on pillow, and diffuse.
Blend: Combine 10 drops cedarwood, 10 drops eucalyptus, 2 drops chamomile (Roman), and 2 oz. water; put on cloth, inhale, or gargle.

ATTACK

Inhale or diffuse bergamot, eucalyptus, hyssop, lavender, or marjoram. Try frankincense for calming.

ASTRINGENT

Lemon

ATHLETE'S FOOT

Cypress, lavender, melaleuca*, myrrh. Blend: Combine 10 drops thyme, 10 drops lavender, 10 drops melaleuca; mix with hand lotion and rub on feet.

ATTENTION DEFICIT DISORDER

(SEE HYPERACTIVE CHILDREN)

Lavender

AWAKE

JET LAG

Eucalyptus, geranium, grapefruit, lavender, lemongrass, peppermint

AWAKEN THE MIND, SPIRIT

Myrrh

AWAKEN THE PAST

Cypress

AWARENESS

Lemongrass

INCREASE AND OPEN SENSORY SYSTEM

Birch

SPIRITUAL

Frankincense, myrrh

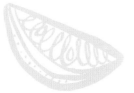

BABIES

All oils used on babies should be diluted. Do Not Use clary sage or spearmint on babies.

BABY OILS
Chamomile (Roman), geranium, lavender

COLIC
Bergamot*, chamomile, fennel, ginger, marjoram*, peppermint.
Blend: Combine 1 drop chamomile (Roman), 1 drop lavender, 1 drop geranium, and 2 Tbls. almond oil. Apply to stomach and back.

COLIC (SEVERE)
Combine 1 drop dill in 1 Tbl. almond oil. Apply to stomach and back.

CRADLE CAP REMEDY
Combine 1 drop eucalyptus, 1 drop lemon, 1 drop geranium, and 2 Tbls. almond oil. Mix and rub on head.

DIAPER RASH
Lavender*
Blend: Combine chamomile, lavender, and birch with pure vegetable oil.

EARACHE
Lavender. Garlic oil works, too, but it is strong smelling,

FRETFUL
Combine 2 drops chamomile, 7 drops tangerine, and 2 Tbls. sweet almond oil; massage baby.

TEETHING
Chamomile

BACK

Basil, birch, chamomile, cypress, eucalyptus, ginger, juniper, lavender, oregano, peppermint, rosemary, sage, thyme (for virus in spine)

CALCIFIED (SPINE)
Geranium, rosemary

HERNIATED DISCS
Cypress (strengthens blood capillary walls, helps with dilation, improves circulation, powerful anti-inflammatory), pepper, peppermint (A compress is good, too.)

LOW BACK PAINS

Massage cypress up the disc area three times. Use helichrysum to increase circulation, decongest, and reduce inflammation and pain. Use peppermint to stimulate the nerves.

MUSCULAR FATIGUE

Clary sage, lavender, marjoram, rosemary

PAIN

Apply the following oils up the spine, one at a time, using a probe on each vertebra if possible. Stroke with fingers, feathering gently in four-inch strokes, three times for each oil: Peppermint (excites the back), cypress (anti-inflammatory), and spruce. Follow the procedure with a hot compress. Blend 5 to 10 drops each rosemary, marjoram, sage.
Blend 5 to 10 drops each lavender, eucalyptus, ginger.
Blend 5 to 10 drops each peppermint, rosemary, basil.

BACTERIA

(SEE ANTIBACTERIAL)

BALANCE

Cedarwood, chamomile, frankincense (balances electrical field), ylang-ylang

MALE/FEMALE ENERGIES

Ylang-ylang

FEELING OF

Spruce

BALDNESS

Cedarwood, rosemary, sage; apply on location and on bottoms of feet.

BATH

Use gentle oils such as chamomile, lavender, rosewood, sage, and ylang-ylang. While tub is filling add oils to the water; oils are drawn to your skin quickly from the top of the water.

BEAUTY

Myrtle (aromatic)

BED-WETTING
(SEE BLADDER)

BEREAVEMENT
Basil, cypress

BIRTHING
(SEE PREGNANCY)

BITES
(SEE INSECT)

Basil, cinnamon, garlic, lavender, lemon, sage, thyme (All have antitoxic and antivenomous properties.)

BEES AND HORNETS
Remove the stinger, apply a cold compress of chamomile to area for several hours or as long as possible. Then apply 1 drop of chamomile three times a day for two days.

GNATS AND MIDGES
Lavender; 3 drops thyme in 1 tsp. cider vinegar or lemon juice; apply to bites to stop irritation.

INSECTS
Patchouly

MOSQUITOS
Helichrysum, lavender

SNAKES
Basil, patchouly

SPIDERS
Mix 3 drops lavender and 2 drops chamomile in 1 tsp. alcohol; mix well clockwise and apply to area three times a day.

SPIDERS, BROWN RECLUSE, BEE STINGS, ANTS, FIRE ANTS
Basil, cinnamon, lavender, lemon, lemongrass, peppermint, thyme

TICKS
After removing tick, apply 1 drop of lavender every 5 minutes, for 30 minutes. To remove: Do not apply mineral oil, Vaseline, or anything else to remove the tick because this may cause it to inject the spirochetes into the wound. Be sure to remove the entire tick. Get as close to the mouth as possible and firmly tug on the tick until it releases its grip. Don't twist. If available, use a magnifying glass to make sure that you remove the entire tick. Save the tick in a jar and label it with the date, where you were

bitten on your body, and the location or address where you were bitten for proper identification by your doctor. Do not handle the tick. Wash hands immediately. Check the site of the bite occasionally to see if any rash develops. If it does, seek medical advice promptly.

WASPS (ARE ALKALINE)

Combine 1 drop basil, 2 drops chamomile, 2 drops lavender, and 1 tsp. cider vinegar; mix clockwise and put on area three times a day.

BITTERNESS

Chamomile

BLADDER

BED-WETTING AND INCONTINENCE

Before bed, rub cypress on abdomen.

INFECTION

Cedarwood, sandalwood (for first stages of infection), lemongrass

BLISTER

ON LIPS (FROM SUN)

Lavender (Apply as often as needed. It should take fever out and return lip to normal.)

BLOOD

Red blood cells carry oxygen throughout the body.

BLOOD TYPES

Different personalities have different dominating glands.

TYPE A

More prone to be alkaline pH balanced. Natural vegetarians. If they eat meat after age 35, they are more prone to get arthritis. Type A child living in a home of type O parent is affected by parent's programing or conditioning or vice versa. They have problems with their thyroid, may have a tendency to gain weight, and need exercise.

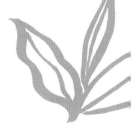

TYPE AB

May want to be a vegetarian some days, but not on others. Can go either way just as A or O types. They may be affected by either the A or O parent.

TYPE B

Down the middle, more balanced. Takes them about three years to convert to being vegetarian.

TYPE O

More prone to acid condition in blood. Big eaters and may need to take more supplements because they are not assimilating the nutrients. If they are not assimilating their food, they eat and get full quickly, and one hour later, they are hungry again. They get more gas because they lack enzyme secretion. They eat more, digest less, but don't gain weight. May take eight years to totally convert to a vegetarian diet. Need more protein; nuts and seeds are a good source. Nutrients in purest form reduce the need to eat. They have a harder time structuring their diet. Get cold because of poor circulation.

BLOOD PRESSURE, HIGH (HYPERTENSION)

Birch*, clary sage, clove, hyssop, lavender, lemon, marjoram, nutmeg, rosemary, spearmint*, ylang-ylang (arterial). Place oils on heart points on left arm, hand, foot, and over heart.

Bath: 3 drops ylang-ylang and 3 drops marjoram in bathwater. Bathe in the evening, twice a week.

Blend #1: 5 drops geranium, 8 drops lemongrass, 3 drops lavender, and 1 oz. pure vegetable oil. Rub over heart and heart reflex on left foot and hand.

Blend #2: 10 drops ylang-ylang, 5 drops marjoram, 5 drops cypress, and 1 oz. pure vegetable oil. Rub over heart and heart reflex on left foot and hand.

LOW

Hyssop (raises), lavender*, marjoram*, rosemary*, ylang-ylang

BLEEDING (STOPS)

Helichrysum, cayenne pepper, rose

BROKEN BLOOD VESSELS

Grapefruit, helichrysum

Tea: Gojo berry

CLEANSING

Camomile, helichrysum. Apply on bottoms of feet.

CLOTS

Grapefruit, helichrysum

HEMORRHAGING *(SEE FEMALE PROBLEMS)*

Helichrysum, rose, cayenne pepper

LOW BLOOD SUGAR

Cinnamon, clove, thyme

STIMULATES

Lemon* helps with the formation of red and white blood cells.

BODY SYSTEMS

Cedarwood

BALANCING

Lavender, spruce

CHEMICALS

Radex (prevents buildup in the body)

CONTROLLING

Cedarwood

ODORS

Sage

RADIATION

Radex (prevents buildup in the body)

STRENGTHEN VITAL CENTERS OF SUPPORT

Oregano, Fir

BOILS

Bergamot, chamomile, clary sage, lavender, lemon, melaleuca

BONES

All the tree oils: birch, cedarwood, fir, juniper, peppermint, sandalwood, spruce.

BONE SPURS

Birch, cypress, marjoram

BROKEN (HEAL)

Blend: 9 drops birch; 8 drops each of spruce, fir, and helichrysum; 7 drops clove (good when inflammation is causing the pain).

BRUISED

Helichrysum

PAIN

Birch

BOREDOM

Cedarwood, chamomile (Roman), cypress, fir, frankincense, juniper, lavender, pepper, rosemary, sandalwood, spruce, thyme, ylang-ylang

BOWEL

IRRITABLE SYNDROME

Peppermint

BRAIN

Clary sage (opens brain, euphoria), cypress, geranium, lemongrass, spearmint

CEREBRAL BRAIN

Nutmeg*

ACTIVATES RIGHT BRAIN

Bergamot, birch, chamomile (Roman), geranium, grapefruit, helichrysum

INJURY

Frankincense; massage on brain stem, diffuse.

INTEGRATION

Clary sage, cypress, geranium, helichrysum, lemongrass, spearmint

TUMOR *(SEE CANCER)*

Frankincense; massage on brain stem, diffuse.

BREAST

Clary sage, cypress, fennel, geranium, lemongrass, sage, spearmint

INCREASE AND FIRM

Clary sage, fennel, sage

BREATHING

Chamomile (Roman), cinnamon, frankincense, ginger, hyssop, juniper, marjoram, nutmeg, rosemary, thyme

HYPERPNEA (ABNORMAL, RAPID BREATHING)

Ylang-ylang*

OXYGEN

Frankincense, sandalwood, all essential oils

BRONCHITIS
(SEE RESPIRATORY SYSTEM)

Bergamot, cedarwood*, chamomile (Roman), clary sage*, clove, cypress, eucalyptus, fir (obstructions of bronchi), frankincense, ginger, lavender, melaleuca*, myrtle*, myrrh, nutmeg, peppermint*, ravensara, rose, rosemary*, sandalwood, spearmint*, thyme*
Blend #1: 10 drops cedarwood and eucalyptus, 2 drops chamomile (Roman), and 2 oz. water; put on cloth, inhale, and gargle.
Blend #2: Clove, cinnamon, melissa, and lavender

CHRONIC

Eucalyptus, ravensara*, sage*, sandalwood*

CLEAR MUCUS

Bergamot, sandalwood, and thyme

IN CHILDREN

Chamomile (Roman), eucalyptus, hyssop, lavender, melaleuca, rosemary, thyme

BRUISES

Fennel, geranium, helichrysum, hyssop, lavender

BUGS (REPEL)
(SEE BITES AND INSECT)

Lemon (kills bugs). Diffuse.

BITES (ALL SPIDERS, BROWN RECLUSE, BEE STINGS, ANTS, FIRE ANTS)

Basil, cinnamon, lavender, lemon, lemongrass, peppermint, thyme

INSECT

Patchouly

SNAKE

Patchouly

BULIMIA

Grapefruit; apply to stomach and bottoms of feet.

BUMPS

Frankincense

BUNIONS

Chamomile (German), carrot oil
Blend: 6 drops eucalyptus, 3 drops lemon, 4 drops ravensara, and 1 drop birch in 1 oz. pure vegetable oil.

BURNS

Chamomile, eucalyptus, geranium, lavender, melaleuca, peppermint, ravensara (healing)
Blend: 10 drops chamomile (blue), 5 drops chamomile (Roman), and 10 drops lavender; mix together and add 1 drop to each square inch of burn after it has been soaked in ice water. If you don't have chamomile, use lavender.

SUNBURN

Melaleuca*

SUNSCREEN

Helichrysum*

BURSITIS

Chamomile (Roman), cypress, ginger, hyssop, juniper
Blend: Apply 6 drops of marjoram on shoulders and arms. Wait 6 minutes, then apply 3 drops of birch. Wait 6 minutes, then apply 3 drops of cypress.

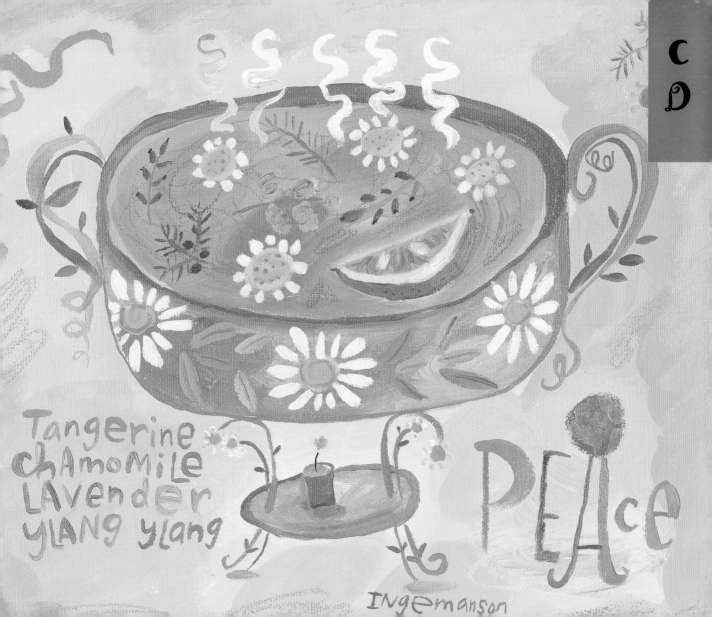

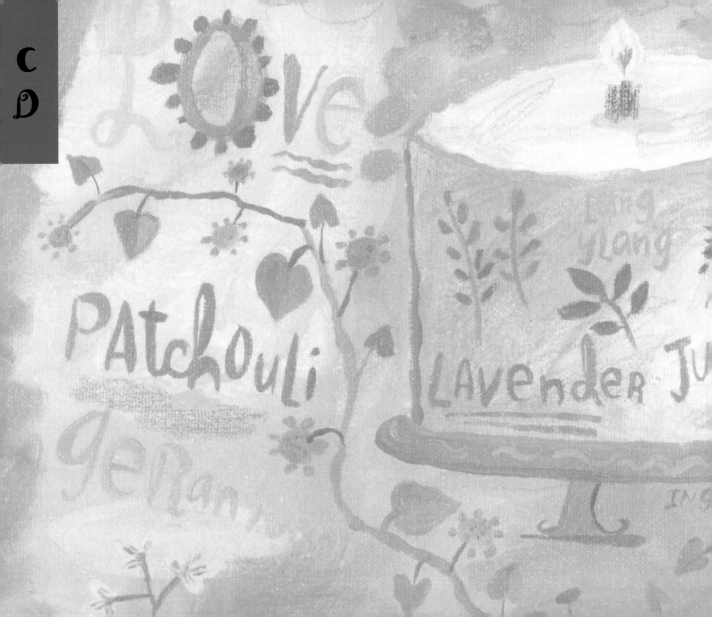

CALCIUM

Carbonated water takes calcium out of the body, blocks potassium, prevents protein absorption, and causes hormone deficiency. Also, when food isn't digested during the night, it ferments and takes oxygen out of the system. When heavy protein is eaten at night, it will not digest by morning.

CALLOUSES

Carrot oil, chamomile, peppermint

CALMING

Bergamot, cedarwood*, clary sage, jasmine, lavender, myrrh, tangerine, ylang-ylang

CANCER
(SEE CHEMICALS)

Clove, frankincense, rose, sage, tarragon* (anticancerous)
Tea: Gojo berry

BONE
Apply frankincense neat.

BRAIN TUMOR
Diffuse frankincense 24 hours a day and massage the brain stem with frankincense.

CERVICAL
Clove, cypress, frankincense, geranium, lavender, lemon

COLON
Diet: Fast 21 days, then have soup (vegetarian). Breakfast: protein foods (vegetarian if possible); lunch: carbohydrates, beans (chile), etc.; nothing but fruits after 3:00 p.m.

LUNG
Blend: 15 drops frankincense, 5 drops clove, 6 drops ravensara, 4 drops myrrh, and 2 drops sage. It is best when inserted into rectum.

LYMPHOMA (NODES OR SMALL TUMORS IN NECK AND GROIN)
Cleanse liver.
Blend 10 drops frankincense, 5 drops myrrh, and 3 drops sage; mix with small amount of pure vegetable oil; apply daily over nodes or tumor areas, and rectally. Every other day apply frankincense, neat.

LYMPHOMA STAGE 4 (BONE MARROW)
Extreme fatigue; eat vegetable and fruits;
no meat.

MELANOMA (SKIN CANCER)
Frankincense and lavender

OVARIAN
Blend: 15 drops frankincense, 6 drops
geranium, 5 drops myrrh, 1/2 tsp. pure
vegetable oil; alternate one night in vagina
(tampon to retain), next night in rectum.

PROSTATE
Fennel, frankincense, sage, yarrow. Apply to
posterior scrotum, ankles, lower back, and
bottoms of feet.

UTERINE
Geranium
Blend: 2 to 5 drops cedarwood or 2 to 5
drops lemon or 2 to 5 drops myrrh in 1 tsp.
pure vegetable oil.

CANDIDA

Cinnamon bark, cloves, eucalyptus*,
melaleuca, mountain savory, neroli,
palmarosa (skin), peppermint (aromatic),
rosemary, rosewood*, spearmint, spruce*,
tarragon (prevents fermentation)

VAGINAL
Bergamot*, melaleuca*, myrrh*

CANKERS
Oregano

CAPILLARIES

BROKEN
Chamomile, cypress, geranium, hyssop
Blend: 1 drop lavender and 1 drop
chamomile; apply.

CARBUNCLES
Melaleuca

CARDIOTONIC
(SEE HEART)

CARDIOVASCULAR SYSTEMS
(SEE HEART)

CARPAL TUNNEL SYNDROME
Eucalyptus, lavender, marjoram

CATARACTS
(SEE EYES)

CATARRH (MUCUS)
(SEE ANTICATARRHAL)
Dill, ginger, myrrh

CAVITIES
(SEE TEETH)

CELIBACY
Marjoram (aromatic)

CELLS
All essential oils restore cells to original state. Need to change the RNA (cell memory) and DNA (cell chemistry) to change the habit.

FREQUENCY
Rose (enhances frequency of every cell, bringing balance and harmony to body)

OXYGENATION
Pepper (black)

REGULATING
Clary sage (removes negative programming)

CELLULITE
(SEE WEIGHT)
Basil, cedarwood*, cypress, fennel, geranium, grapefruit*, juniper, lemon, orange, oregano, patchouly, rosemary, rosewood*, sage, tangerine (dissolves), thyme

ATTACKS FAT
Basil, grapefruit, lavender, lemongrass, rosemary, sage, thyme

CHAKRAS (BALANCES)

Lavender (brings harmony to chakras), sandalwood (affects each chakra differently), helichrysum (unites head and heart)

CROWN

Sandalwood

BROW (THIRD EYE)

Juniper, peppermint, rosemary, frankincense (opens)

THROAT

Sandalwood

HEART

Sandalwood, bergamot (opens)

SOLAR PLEXUS

Fennel, juniper

SACRAL (NAVEL)

Patchouly, sandalwood, sage (balancing)

BASE

Patchouly, sandalwood

CHEEKS

Jasmine

CHICKEN POX
(SEE CHILDHOOD DISEASES)

CHILDBIRTH
(SEE PREGNANCY)

CHILDHOOD DISEASES

CHICKEN POX (2 WEEKS) (SEE SHINGLES)

Sleep is very good. Bergamot, chamomile, eucalyptus, lavender, melaleuca (tea tree) Bath: Combine 2 drops lavender, 1 cup bicarbonate of soda, and 1 cup soda in bath and soak. Relieves itching.
Blend #1: Combine 10 drops lavender, 10 drops chamomile, 4 oz. calamine lotion; mix and apply twice a day all over body. Or 5 to 10 drops each of chamomile (German) and lavender to 1 oz. calamine lotion.
Blend #2: Combine 10 drops lavender, 10 drops chamomile (blue), and 4 oz. calamine lotion. Mix and apply twice a day all over body.

MEASLES

Chamomile, eucalyptus*, lavender, melaleuca. Spray or vaporize room.

GERMAN (3-DAY)

Treat in same way as viral infections.

RUBELLA

Sponge with one of these oils: Chamomile (Roman or German), lavender, melaleuca.

MUMPS

Lavender, lemon, melaleuca

WHOOPING COUGH

Cinnamon, clary sage, cypress, grapefruit, hyssop, lavender, oregano*, thyme

CHILDREN

(SEE BABIES, HYPERACTIVE CHILDREN, CHILDHOOD DISEASES)

CHILLS

Ginger. Apply on bottoms of feet and on solar plexus.

CHOLERA

Clove, ravensara*, rosemary*

CHOLESTEROL

Clary sage*, helichrysum* (regulates); apply on heart and along arms.
Tea: Gojo berry

CIGARETTES

(SEE ADDICTIONS)

CIRCULATION

Birch, cinnamon bark, clary sage, cypress*, hyssop, nutmeg
Tea: Gojo berry

CIRCULATORY SYSTEM

Clary sage, cypress, helichrysum, nutmeg* (stimulant)

CIRRHOSIS

(SEE LIVER)

CLARITY OF THOUGHT
Rosemary

CLEANSING
Fennel, juniper, melaleuca (aromatic)

CUTS
Lavender

COCKROACHES
Blend 10 drops peppermint, 5 drops cypress, 1/2 cup water, and spray.

COLDS
Eucalyptus (in hot water, breathe deep), fir (aches and pain), ginger, lavender, lemon*, melaleuca*, myrtle, orange, oregano, peppermint*, ravensara, rosemary*, thyme, wild tansy

COLD SORES
(SEE HERPES SIMPLEX)
Bergamot, melaleuca

COLIC
(SEE BABIES)

COLITIS
Clove (bacterial), helichrysum* (when it's viral), tarragon*, diatomaceous earth (Redmond clay) to get into pockets in the colon, thyme* (when there is infection)

COLON
(SEE COLITIS AND DIVERTICULITIS)
Use diatomaceous earth (Redmond clay) to get into the pockets of the colon.

COMPASSION
Helichrysum (promotes)

COMPLEXION

(SEE SKIN)

Apply oils to face, neck, and intestines.

DULL

Jasmine

OILY

Orange

CONCENTRATION (POOR)

Basil, cedarwood, cypress, eucalyptus, juniper, lavender, lemon, myrrh, orange, peppermint, rosemary, sandalwood, ylang-ylang

CONCUSSION

Cypress. Rub on brain stem and bottoms of feet.

CONFIDENCE

Jasmine, sandalwood

CONFUSION

Basil, cedarwood, cypress, fir, frankincense, geranium, ginger, jasmine, juniper, marjoram, peppermint, rose, rosemary, rosewood, sandalwood, spruce, thyme, ylang-ylang

CONGESTION

Cedarwood, ginger. To help discharge mucus, rub oil(s) on chest, neck, back, feet, and diffuse.

CONSCIOUSNESS

Lavender (aromatic)

OPEN

Rosemary (aromatic)

PURIFYING

Peppermint (aromatic)

STIMULATING

Peppermint (aromatic)

CONSTIPATION

Fennel, ginger, juniper, marjoram*, orange*, patchouly, pepper (black), rose, rosemary, sandalwood, tangerine, tarragon; massage clockwise around abdomen.
Blend #1: Mix together 6 drops of orange*, tangerine, and spearmint, and rub on lower stomach and colon.
Blend #2: Combine 15 drops cedarwood, 10 drops lemon, 5 drops peppermint, and 2 oz. pure vegetable oil. Massage clockwise over lower abdomen three times a day and take supplements.

CHILDREN

Fruit juices, lots of water, chamomile (Roman), geranium, patchouly, rosemary, tangerine

CONTAGIOUS DISEASES

Ginger

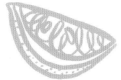

CONTROL

OF YOUR LIFE

Cedarwood

SELF

Chamomile (aromatic)

CONVULSIONS

Chamomile, clary sage, lavender

COOLING OILS

Chamomile (Roman), eucalyptus, lavender, melaleuca, peppermint

CORNS

Carrot, chamomile, lemon, peppermint

CORTISONE

Birch, chamomile, lavender, spruce* (like cortisone)
Blend: Combine 3 drops chamomile, 3 drops lavender, 5 drops spruce, and 1 drop birch; apply as a natural cortisone.

COUGHS

Chamomile, cedarwood, eucalyptus*, fir, frankincense, ginger, jasmine, juniper, melaleuca*, myrtle*, myrrh, peppermint, myrrh, ravensara, sandalwood, thyme

BAD

Blend: 3 drops fir, 3 drops lemon, 2 drops ravensara, 1 drop thyme, 1 tsp. honey.

SMOKER'S

Myrtle

COURAGE

Clove (aromatic), fennel (aromatic), ginger

CRADLE CAP

(SEE BABIES)

CRAMPS

Basil, birch*, cypress*, ginger, lavender*, rosemary, marjoram*

CROHN'S DISEASE

Basil

CUTS

(SEE TISSUE)

Chamomile (healing), cypress, helichrysum, lavender, melaleuca, ravensara, rosewood

CYSTITIS (BLADDER INFECTION)

Basil, bergamot, cedarwood, chamomile, cinnamon, clove, eucalyptus, fennel*, frankincense, hyssop, juniper, lavender, marjoram, oregano, sage, sandalwood, rosewood, thyme*; massage or bathe with one of these oils.

DANDRUFF

Cedarwood, lavender*, melaleuca, patchouly, rosemary, sage

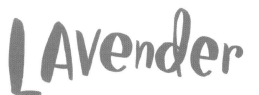

DAYDREAMING

Cedarwood, eucalyptus, ginger, helichrysum, lavender, lemon, myrrh, peppermint, rose, rosemary, rosewood, sandalwood, spruce, thyme, ylang-ylang

DEBILITY

Nutmeg*

DECONGESTANT

Chamomile (blue), citrus oils, cypress*, juniper, melaleuca, and patchouly

DEGENERATIVE DISEASE

(SEE SPECIFIC AILMENT)

All essential oils.

DELIVERY

(SEE PREGNANCY)

DENIAL

Chamomile, sage

DENTAL INFECTION

Clove and frankincense, helichrysum, melaleuca, myrrh; apply to jaws and gums.

DEODORIZING

Clary sage, myrrh*, peppermint, sage, thyme

DEPLETION

Cypress

DEPRESSION

Bergamot (aromatic), chamomile (Roman), clary sage, frankincense, geranium, ginger, grapefruit, jasmine, juniper (over heart), lavender (aromatic), patchouly, pepper (on crown for spirit protection), rosewood*, sage (relieves depression), sandalwood, tangerine, ylang-ylang*

ANTIDEPRESSANT

Bergamot, chamomile, frankincense, geranium, jasmine, lavender, melissa, rose

IMMUNE DEPRESSION

Spruce*
Blend: 5 drops bergamot, 5 drops lavender, diffuse

SEDATIVES

Chamomile, clary sage, sandalwood, ylang-ylang

CLEANSING FLESH AND BLOOD OF EVIL DEITIES

Cedarwood and myrrh

DERMATITIS

Bergamot, chamomile (blue and German), geranium, helichrysum*, hyssop, juniper*, lavender, patchouly*, thyme*

DESPAIR

Cedarwood, clary sage, fir, frankincense, geranium, lavender, lemon, lemongrass, orange, peppermint, rosemary, sandalwood, spearmint, spruce, thyme, ylang-ylang

DESPONDENCY

Bergamot, clary sage, cypress, geranium, ginger, orange, rose, rosewood, sandalwood, and ylang-ylang

DETOXIFICATION

Helichrysum*, juniper* (detoxifier). Apply oils to liver area and intestines.

DIABETES

(Watch insulin intake carefully; may have to cut down.) Coriander (normalizes glucose levels), cypress, dill (helps lower glucose levels by normalizing insulin levels and supporting pancreas function), Eucalyptus*, fennel, geranium*, ginger, hyssop, juniper, lavender, rosemary*, ylang-ylang*

Blend #1: 8 drops clove, 8 drops cinnamon bark, 15 drops rosemary, 10 drops thyme in 2 oz. of pure vegetable oil. Put on feet and over pancreas.

Blend #2: 5 drops cinnamon and cypress. Rub on feet and pancreas.

Tea: Gojo berry (prevents)

PANCREAS SUPPORT

Cinnamon, fennel, geranium

DIAPER RASH

Lavender*

DIARRHEA

Geranium*, ginger*, melaleuca, myrrh*, myrtle, peppermint*, sandalwood*, spearmint (not for babies)

ANTISPASMODIC

Chamomile, cypress, eucalyptus

CHILDREN

Chamomile (Roman), geranium, ginger, sandalwood

CHRONIC

Nutmeg*, orange*

STRESS-INDUCED

Lavender

DIET

POST-DIET SAGGY SKIN

Combine 8 drops sage, 8 drops lemongrass, and 1 oz. pure vegetable oil. Rub on areas.

DIGESTIVE SYSTEM
(SEE INTESTINAL PROBLEMS)

Black cumin, cinnamon bark, clary sage (weak), fennel (sluggish), ginger, grapefruit, juniper, lemon (indigestion), lemongrass (purifier), mandarin (tonic), marjoram* (stimulates), myrrh, neroli, nutmeg (for sluggishness; eases digestion), orange (indigestion), patchouly, pepper (black), peppermint, rosemary, sage* (sluggish), spearmint, tangerine (nervous and sluggish), tarragon (nervous and sluggish). Add the oil(s) to your food, rub on stomach, or apply as a compress over abdomen.

DISAPPOINTMENT

Clary sage, eucalyptus, fir, frankincense, geranium, ginger, juniper, lavender, orange, spruce, thyme, ylang-ylang

DISCOURAGEMENT

Bergamot, cedarwood, frankincense, geranium, juniper, lavender, lemon, orange, rosewood, sandalwood, spruce

DISINFECTANT

Grapefruit, lemon*, sage*
Add the following number of drops to a bowl of water: 10 lavender (2), 20 thyme (4), 5 eucalyptus (1), 5 oregano (1). If using the larger portions, add to a large bowl of water. If using the amounts in parentheses, add to a small bowl of water. Use to disinfect small areas.

DIURETIC

Cedarwood*, cypress, fennel, grapefruit (all citrus oils), juniper, lavender*, lemon, lemongrass*, marjoram, orange, oregano, rosemary*, sage*; apply oil(s) to kidney area on back, bottoms of feet, and on location.

ALLEVIATE FLUIDS

Cypress, fennel, tangerine
Blend: Combine 1 drop fennel, 2 drops cypress, 5 drops tangerine; apply from the top of the foot to the knee.

DIVERTICULITIS

Diatomaceous earth (Redmond clay) to get into pockets. Rub abdomen with cinnamon and pure vegetable oil. Lavender.

DIZZINESS

Tangerine

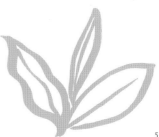

DNA

Chamomile strengthens positive imprinting in DNA.

DROWNING IN OWN NEGATIVITY

Grapefruit (prevent, aromatic)

DRUGS
(SEE ADDICTIONS)

DYSENTERY

Chamomile, clove (amebic), cypress, eucalyptus, lemon, melissa, myrrh*, pepper (black); apply on abdomen and bottoms of feet.

DYSPEPSIA (IMPAIRED DIGESTION)

Tarragon, grapefruit*, myrrh, orange (nervous), thyme*; apply to stomach and intestines.

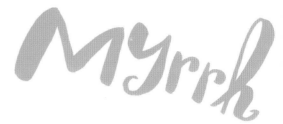

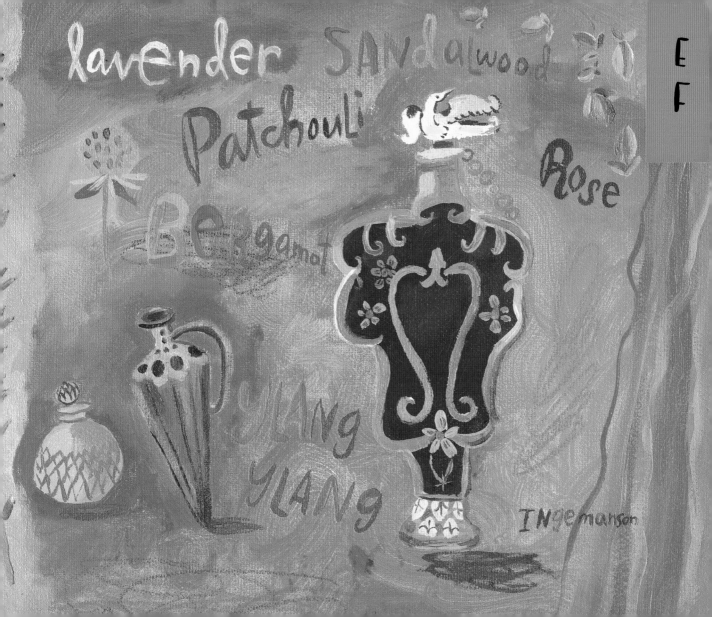

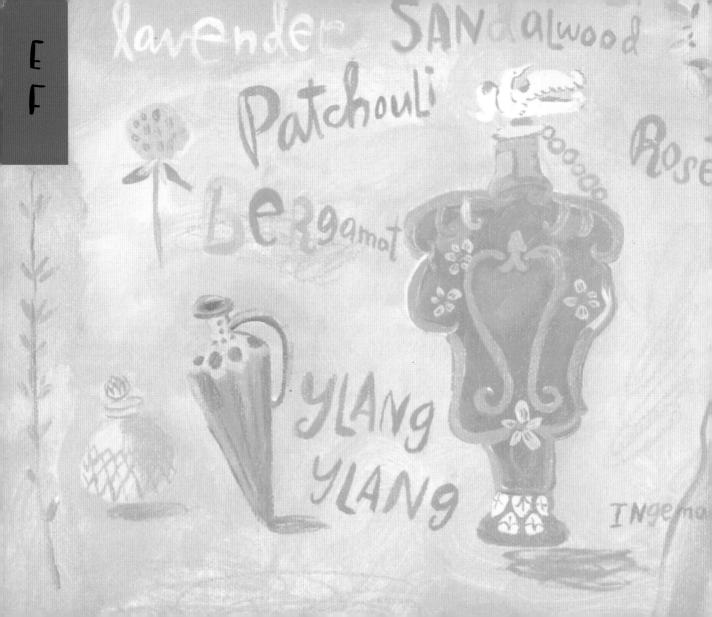

EARS

Eucalyptus, geranium, helichrysum, juniper

INCREASE AND RESTORE HEARING

Rub 1 drop helichrysum around inside of ear with finger. Not deep in ear. Then do the following ear adjustment: Pull one ear up, then the other ear up, 10 times each side. Pull one ear back, then the other, 5 times each side. Pull one ear down, then the other, 5 times each side. Pull one ear forward, then the other, 5 times each side. Then one quick pull in each direction. Up, back, down, forward.

Rub juniper all around, back and front of ear. Rub geranium all around, back and front of ear.

INFECTION

Melaleuca, lavender (all around outside of ear)

INFLAMMATION

Eucalyptus

TINNITUS (RINGING IN EARS, BLOCK IN EUSTACHIAN TUBE)

Helichrysum (rub on inside and outside of ears), juniper

EATING DISORDERS

ANOREXIA

Grapefruit

BULIMIA

Grapefruit

OVEREATING

Ginger, lemon, peppermint, spearmint

ECZEMA

Bergamot, chamomile, eucalyptus, helichrysum*, juniper*, lavender, melissa, patchouly*, rosewood*, sage

DRY

Bergamot, chamomile, geranium, hyssop, rosemary

WET

Chamomile, hyssop, juniper, lavender, myrrh

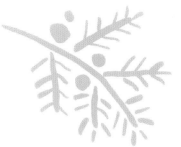

EDEMA

(SEE HORMONAL IMBALANCE)

Cypress* (alleviates fluids), fennel (breaks up fluids), juniper, geranium, lemongrass*, rosemary, tangerine (alleviates fluids)
Blend: 1 drop fennel, 2 drops cypress, 5 drops tangerine; apply from the top of the foot to the knee.

ANKLES

Combine 5 drops cypress, 3 drops juniper, and 10 drops tangerine; apply from ankles to knees.

DIURETIC

Cedarwood*, cypress, fennel, grapefruit, juniper, lavender*, lemon, lemongrass*, orange, oregano, rosemary*, sage*

ELBOW

(SEE TENNIS ELBOW)

ELEVATING THE BODY

Birch, all high-vibration oils

EMOTIONS

Blue chamomile (stability), cypress (aromatic, healing)

BLOCKS

Spearmint and spruce help to release emotional blocks.

CLEARING

Juniper

COLDNESS (EMOTIONAL)

Myrrh, ylang-ylang

CONFIDENCE

Jasmine (euphoria)

EASE FEELING OF LOSS

Tangerine (stability)

EMOTIONAL TRAUMA

Sandalwood

GRIEF

Tangerine (aromatic; increases optimism and releases emotional stress)

EMPHYSEMA

Eucalyptus

ENDOCRINE SYSTEM

Cinnamon bark, dill, pepper (black), rosemary*

ENDOMETRIOSIS

(SEE HORMONAL IMBALANCE)

Clary sage, cypress, eucalyptus, geranium, nutmeg

ENERGY

Basil (when squandering energy), cypress, eucalyptus (builds), fir*, juniper, lemon, nutmeg (increases), orange (aromatic), pepper (black), peppermint, rosemary, thyme (aromatic—gives energy in times of physical weakness and stress)

INCREASE

Eucalyptus, grapefruit, peppermint, rosemary

INTEGRATE FOR EQUAL DISTRIBUTION

Patchouly

NEGATIVE

Ginger and juniper (clear negative energy)

PHYSICAL

Bergamot, cinnamon bark (aromatic), lemon (aromatic), patchouly (aromatic)

SEXUAL

Ylang-ylang (aromatic; influences)

ENLIGHTENING

Helichrysum

EQUILIBRIUM

Ylang-ylang

NERVE

Petitgrain

ESSENTIAL OILS

CAUSTIC, NEED TO DILUTE

Cinnamon, clove fennel, grapefruit, lemon, nutmeg, orange, oregano, peppermint; dilute 1 drop of oil to 20 drops lavender or mix with pure vegetable oil.

ESTROGEN

Clary sage (helps body to produce)

EUPHORIA

Clary sage (aromatic), jasmine

EXHAUSTION

First, use the following nervous system oils to calm and relax: Bergamot, chamomile (Roman), clary sage, frankincense, or lavender. Second, use basil, ginger, grapefruit, lavender, lemon, rosemary, or sandalwood.

EXPECTORANT

Eucalyptus, frankincense, helichrysum, marjoram*, pepper (black), and ravensara; apply to throat, lungs, and diffuse.

EYES

Chamomile (German), cypress (also helps circulation), fennel, frankincense, lavender, lemon, lemongrass (improves eyesight) Base oils (good blends of): Almond or hazelnut

CATARACTS

Blend: 8 drops lemongrass, 6 drops cypress, and 3 drops eucalyptus. Apply around the eye area two times a day. Don't get in the eyes.

DRY, ITCHY

Melaleuca (in humidifier)

EYELID DROP

Helichrysum and peppermint (don't get in eyes)

IMPROVE VISION

Frankincense, juniper, lemongrass; apply oils to feet, thumbs, ankles, pelvis, eye area (not in eyes), eyebrows
Blend #1: 10 drops lemongrass, 5 drops cypress, 3 drops eucalyptus; apply around eyes morning and night.
Blend #2: 5 drops lemongrass, 3 drops cypress, 2 drops eucalyptus, and 1 oz. pure vegetable oil. Apply as a blend or layer the oils on the eye area (not in eyes).

IRIS, INFLAMMATION OF

Eucalyptus

RETINA, BLEEDING IN

Blend: 5 drops tangerine, 5 drops orange, and 5 drops grapefruit; mix and apply 2 drops on fingers and toes. Diffuse and let vapor mist around eye. Then, eat two whole oranges a day with the white still on the orange. Eat all the white you can.

STRENGTHEN

Peppermint, lavender, lemongrass, helichrysum. Apply oil(s) around eye area. Blend: 5 drops juniper, 3 drops lemongrass, 3 drops cypress. Rub on brain stem twice a day.

SWOLLEN EYES

Cypress and helichrysum; lavender (antiseptic) is also safe around eyes. If due to allergies, try putting peppermint on the back of the neck.

FACIAL OILS

BROKEN CAPILLARIES

Chamomile, cypress, geranium, hyssop

DEHYDRATED

Geranium, lavender

DISTURBED

Chamomile, clary sage, geranium, hyssop, juniper, lavender, lemon, patchouly, sandalwood

DRY

Chamomile (blue), geranium, hyssop, lemon, patchouly, rosemary, sandalwood

ENERGIZING

Bergamot, lemon

HYDRATED

Cypress, fennel, geranium, hyssop, lavender, lemon, patchouly, sandalwood

NORMAL

Chamomile, geranium, lavender, lemon, sandalwood

OILY

Chamomile, cypress, frankincense, geranium, jasmine, juniper, lavender, lemon, marjoram, orange, patchouly, rosemary

REVITALIZING

Cypress, fennel, lemon

SENSITIVE

Chamomile (blue), geranium, lavender

FAINTING
(SEE SHOCK)

Nutmeg. Hold one of the following under the nose: Basil, lavender, pepper (black), peppermint, rosemary.

FAT
(SEE CELLULITE AND WEIGHT)

Blend: 8 drops grapefruit, 5 drops cypress, 4 drops lavender, 4 drops basil, and 3 drops juniper. Bath (attack fat): Add 6 drops of blend to bathwater and soak in tub.
Tea: Gojo berry

FATIGUE

Clove, ravensara*, rosemary, thyme* (general)

MENTAL

Basil; apply on temples, back of neck, feet, and diffuse.

OVERCOMING

Thyme, on spine

FATTY DEPOSITS
(SEE CELLULITE AND WEIGHT)

FEAR

Bergamot, chamomile (Roman), clary sage, cypress, fir, geranium, juniper, marjoram, myrrh, orange, sandalwood, spruce, rose, ylang-ylang

FEET

Chamomile, fennel, lavender, lemon

CALLOUSES *(SEE CALLOUSES)*

CLUB FOOT

Massage with one of the following: Chamomile, ginger, lavender, rosemary. (Ginger and rosemary not to be used on babies except for club foot.)

CORNS *(SEE CORNS)*

Lemon

ODOR

Mix 1 Tbl. baking powder with 2 drops of sage and put in a plastic bag. Shake, eliminate lumps (with rolling pin), and sprinkle in shoes.

FEMALE PROBLEMS

Clary Sage

(SEE HORMONAL IMBALANCE, INFERTILITY, MENOPAUSE, MENSTRUAL, OVARIES, PMS, PREGNANCY, UTERUS, ETC.)

BALANCE HORMONES

Bergamot, ylang-ylang

CRAMPS *(SEE CRAMPS)*

HEMORRHAGING *(SEE HEMORRHAGING)*

INFECTION

Bergamot* (general)

INFERTILITY (FEMALE)

Chamomile (Roman), clary sage, cypress, fennel, geranium, nutmeg, thyme

POSTPARTUM DEPRESSION

Nutmeg

FEVER

Eucalyptus*, fennel (breaks up), fir, ginger, lavender, lemon (reduces), melaleuca, peppermint* (diffuse), spearmint (not on babies)

TO COOL SYSTEM

Bergamot, eucalyptus, peppermint

TO INDUCE SWEATING

Basil, chamomile, cypress, fennel, lavender, melaleuca, peppermint, rosemary

FIBROCYSTS
(SEE HORMONAL IMBALANCE)

FIBROIDS
(SEE HORMONAL IMBALANCE)

Lavender, frankincense; put 3 drops of either oil in douche.

FIBROMYALGIA
(SEE HORMONAL IMBALANCE)

Use the anti-inflammatory oils: Birch, helichrysum, lavender, myrrh, patchouly, rosemary, rosewood, spruce, thyme.

FIBROSITIS

(SEE HORMONAL IMBALANCE)

Blend: Combine 2 drops cinnamon bark, 10 drops eucalyptus, 10 drops ginger, 6 drops nutmeg, 10 drops peppermint, and 3 drops rosemary with 2 Tbls. pure vegetable oil and massage chest and back once a day.

FINGER

MASHED

Geranium (for bruising), helichrysum (to stop the bleeding), lavender (general healing), lemongrass (for tissue repair)

FLATULENCE (GAS)

Bergamot, chamomile, coriander, eucalyptus, fennel*, ginger*, juniper, lavender*, myrrh, nutmeg, peppermint, rosemary, spearmint (not for babies), tarragon*; apply to stomach and abdomen.

FLU

Clove, eucalyptus, fir (aches and pains), ginger, lavender, melaleuca*, myrtle*, orange, peppermint*, rosemary, thyme (apply to feet; apply where flu has settled), wild tansy

FLUIDS

(SEE EDEMA OR DIURETIC)

FORGETFULNESS

Cedarwood, chamomile (Roman), cypress, fir, geranium, juniper, marjoram, myrrh, orange, rose, sandalwood, rose, ylang-ylang

FORTIFYING

Cypress

FRIGIDITY

Clary sage*, jasmine, nutmeg (overcome and impotency), rose, ylang-ylang*

FRUSTRATION

Chamomile (Roman), clary sage,
frankincense, ginger, juniper, lavender,
lemon, orange, peppermint, spruce, thyme,
ylang-ylang

FUNGUS

Chamomile, cloves, fennel, melaleuca
Blend: 2 drops myrrh and 2 drops lavender;
put on location.

FUNGAL INFECTION

Geranium, melaleuca, patchouly

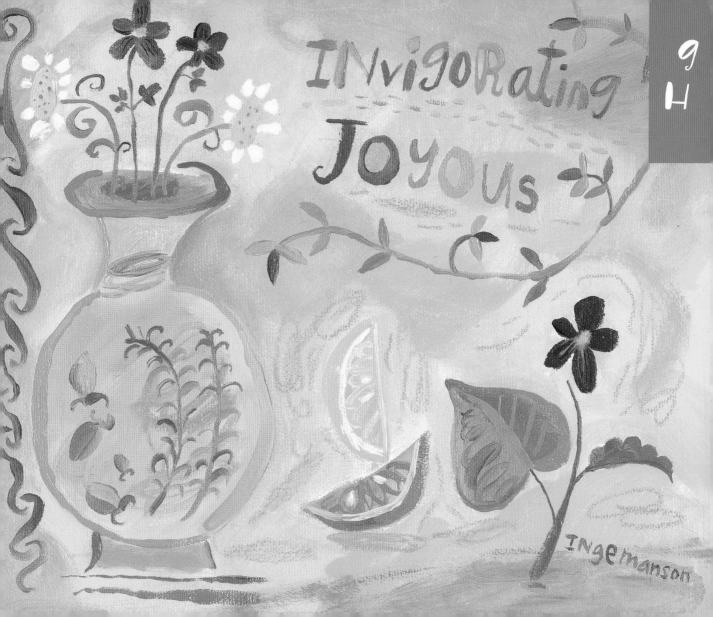

INviGORating

JOYOUS

9
H

Ingemanson

GALLBLADDER

Geranium, juniper, lavender; apply to gallbladder area.

INFECTION

Helichrysum*

STONES

Grapefruit, nutmeg*

GAS

(SEE FLATULENCE)

Lavender*, nutmeg, tarragon

GASTRITIS

Sage*

GENERAL TONIC

Grapefruit, lemon, mountain savory, spruce*

GENITALS

Clary sage*

GENTLENESS

Rosewood (aromatic)

GERMS

(SEE BACTERIA)

AIRBORNE

Fir

GERMICIDAL

Lemon*

GINGIVITIS

Helichrysum, melaleuca, myrrh, rose, rosemary; apply on throat and gums.

GLANDULAR SYSTEM

Sage*, spearmint, spruce

GOUT

Basil, birch, fennel*, hyssop, lemon*, nutmeg, thyme

Grief/Sorrow

Bergamot (turns grief into joy), chamomile (Roman), clary sage, eucalyptus, juniper, lavender

Grounding

Fir, patchouly, spruce

FEELING OF

Cypress (aromatic)

Guilt

Chamomile (Roman), cypress, frankincense, geranium, juniper, lemon, marjoram, rose, sandalwood, spruce, thyme

Gum Disease

Melaleuca*, myrrh

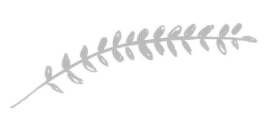

Gums

Chamomile (Roman), lavender

INFECTION

Myrrh

SURGERY ON GUMS

Helichrysum applied with a Q-tip every 15 minutes to kill pain.

Habits

(SEE ADDICTIONS)

Lavender

Hair

BEARD

Cypress, lavender, lemon, rosemary, thyme

CARE

Chamomile

COLOR (KEEP LIGHT)

Combine 1 drop Chamomile, 1 drop lemon, and 1 quart water. Rinse hair.

DANDRUFF

Basil, birch, cedarwood, cypress, lavender*, rosemary, sage, thyme

DRY

Birch, geranium, lavender, rosemary, sandalwood

FRAGILE HAIR

Birch, chamomile, clary sage, lavender, sandalwood, thyme

GROWTH (STIMULATE)

Basil, cedarwood, cypress, geranium, ginger, grapefruit, hyssop, lavender, lemon, rosemary, sage, thyme, ylang-ylang (promotes)

ITCHING

Lavender and peppermint* (skin)

LOSS

Birch, cedarwood, chamomile (Roman), clary sage, cypress, lavender*, lemon, rosemary*, sage, thyme, ylang-ylang*
Blend: Combine 2 drops cinnamon bark, 4 drops cypress, 4 drops geranium, 2 drops juniper, 5 drops lavender, and 3 drops rosemary. Put one drop into 1/4 tsp. of water and rub on bald area and entire scalp. A gentle night treatment.

HALITOSIS

Cardamon, lavender, nutmeg*, peppermint

HANDS

Eucalyptus, geranium, lavender, lemon, patchouly, rosemary, sandalwood

DRY, NEGLECTED

Geranium, patchouly, sandalwood

HANGOVER

Fennel, grapefruit, lavender, lemon, rose, rosemary, sandalwood

HARMONY IN BODY SYSTEMS

Chamomile, clove (aromatic), geranium (harmonizing)

HARSHNESS

Jasmine

HAY FEVER

Chamomile, eucalyptus, lavender, melissa, rose

HEADACHES

Clove, eucalyptus, frankincense, lavender, marjoram, peppermint*, rosemary*; apply to temples, back of neck, forehead, and diffuse.

CHILDREN'S MIGRAINES

Blend 5 drops Chamomile, 10 drops grapefruit, 5 drops peppermint, 3 drops rosemary, and 4 oz. pure vegetable oil for children under seven, and 2 oz. pure vegetable oil for children over seven.

MENSTRUAL MIGRAINES *(SEE HORMONE IMBALANCE)*

MIGRAINES

Basil, birch, chamomile, marjoram, peppermint*, spearmint, ylang-ylang

STRESS

Chamomile

HEALING

Clary sage (aromatic), clove, cypress, eucalyptus (aromatic), frankincense, lemon (aromatic), melaleuca, sage

HEALTH

Lavender (aromatic), lemon (aromatic)

PROMOTES

Eucalyptus, juniper (aromatic)

HEARING

(SEE EARS)

HEART

Cypress, geranium, ginger, hyssop, lavender, rosemary, ylang-ylang (balances heart function). Apply oils to carotids, heart, feet, under left ring finger, above elbow, and behind ring toe on left foot.

CARDIOTONIC

Lavender, thyme

CARDIOVASCULAR SYSTEM

Cinnamon bark (strengthening), fennel, orange* (cardiac spasms), palmarosa (supports), sandalwood (strengthens)

HEART PUMP

Using the thumbs, pump, alternating between the following two points: (1) on the left hand at the lifeline under the ring finger, and (2) just inside the elbow (heart point).

HYPERTENSION *(SEE BLOOD)*

IRREGULAR

Lavender

PALPITATIONS

Lavender, melissa, orange*, peppermint, ylang-ylang*

STRENGTHEN HEART MUSCLE

Lavender, marjoram, peppermint, rose, rosemary

STRENGTHENING (GENERAL)

Cinnamon bark

TACHYCARDIA

Lavender*, orange*

HEARTBURN

Lemon*, peppermint* (over thymus) Blend: 2 drops lemon, 2 drops peppermint, 3 drops sandalwood, and 1/2 oz. pure vegetable oil. Apply to breastbone. Using palm of hand, massage in a clockwise motion applying pressure.

HEMATOMA (SWELLING OR TUMOR FILLED WITH DIFFUSED BLOOD)

Chamomile (blue), helichrysum*

HEMORRHAGING

Helichrysum, rose, ylang-ylang. Massage around ankles, lower back, and stomach. Cayenne pepper may also help.

HEMORRHOIDS

Basil, clary sage*, cypress*, frankincense, helichrysum, juniper, myrrh, patchouly*, peppermint*; put cypress and helichrysum inside on location.

HEPATITIS

Chamomile, cinnamon, cypress, eucalyptus, melaleuca, oregano, patchouly, rosemary, thyme

VIRAL

Myrrh*, ravensara*, rosemary; apply to spine and liver area.

HERNIA

Apply oil(s) on location and lower back.

HIATAL HERNIA

Basil, cypress, fennel, geranium, ginger, hyssop, lavender, peppermint, rosemary

INCISIONAL HERNIA

Basil, geranium, ginger, helichrysum, lavender, lemon, lemongrass, melaleuca

INGUINAL

Lavender, lemongrass

HERPES SIMPLEX

Lavender*, ravensara*

HICCUPS

Sandalwood, tarragon*

HIGH BLOOD PRESSURE

(SEE BLOOD)

HIVES

(SEE pH BALANCE)

Hives may be the result of too much acid in the blood. Patchouly may relieve itching. Chamomile.

HODGKIN'S DISEASE

Clove. Apply to liver and kidney.

HORMONAL IMBALANCE

A hormonal imbalance can cause many problems, including PMS, pre- and post-menopausal conditions, depression, endometriosis, fibromyalgia, fibrocysts, infertility, insomnia, irregular menstrual cycles, lowered libido, menstrual migraines, osteoporosis, ovarian cysts, unexplained first-trimester miscarriage, water retention, etc. It is often a result of estrogen dominance; that is, there is not enough progesterone to balance the amount of estrogen. Estrogen is manufactured in several places in the body and is also found in much of our food, especially animal and dairy products. However, there is only one place in a woman's body where progesterone is produced and that is in the ovaries. If the ovaries are not functioning properly, have been removed, or if they have atrophied because of menopause or hysterectomy, the woman is undoubtedly estrogen dominant and therefore a candidate for these problems. One successful treatment is natural progesterone (obtained from the wild yam). A good book to read about this is entitled *Natural Progesterone: The Multiple Roles of a Remarkable Hormone*, by Dr. John R. Lee, M.D. To obtain a copy, you may write to Connie Higley at 11569 S. Burch Circle, Olathe, KS 66061, or call (913) 438-2957.

HORMONAL SYSTEM

Davana, sandalwood* (hormonelike), spearmint*

BALANCE FEMALE

Bergamot, nutmeg, ylang-ylang

BALANCE

Bergamot, clary sage*, clove (aromatic), fennel, geranium, nutmeg, sage, ylang-ylang

SEXUAL ENERGY

Ylang-ylang

HOT FLASHES

(SEE HORMONAL IMBALANCE)

Bergamot (estrogen), clary sage (estrogen), fennel, or peppermint*; apply these oils on the ankles.

HOUSECLEANING

Fir, lemon, or spruce work well for polishing furniture and cleaning and disinfecting bathrooms and kitchens. Put a few drops on your dust cloth or put 10 drops in water in a spray bottle to spray as a mist. Lemon oil is terrific for dissolving gum and grease.

DISHES

A couple of drops of lemon in the dishwater make dishes sparkle and the kitchen smell great.

LAUNDRY

Adding oils to washer can increase antibacterial benefits; clothes come out with refreshing, clean smell.

HYPERACTIVE CHILDREN

Chamomile (Roman), lavender; diffuse

HYPERPNEA (ABNORMAL, RAPID BREATHING)

Ylang ylang*; apply to lung area.

HYPERTENSION

(SEE BLOOD, HIGH BLOOD PRESSURE)

HYPOGLYCEMIA

Cinnamon bark, clove, eucalyptus, thyme

HYSTERIA

Lavender, melaleuca; apply to heart, bottom of feet, and diffuse.

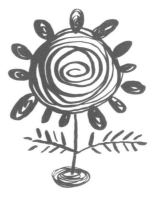

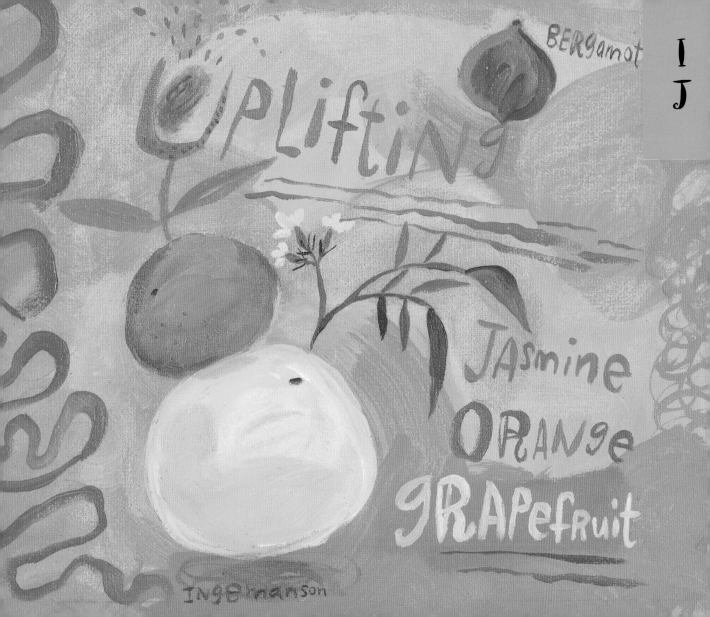

Uplifting

BERGamot

I
J

Jasmine
ORANge
gRApefruit

INgermanson

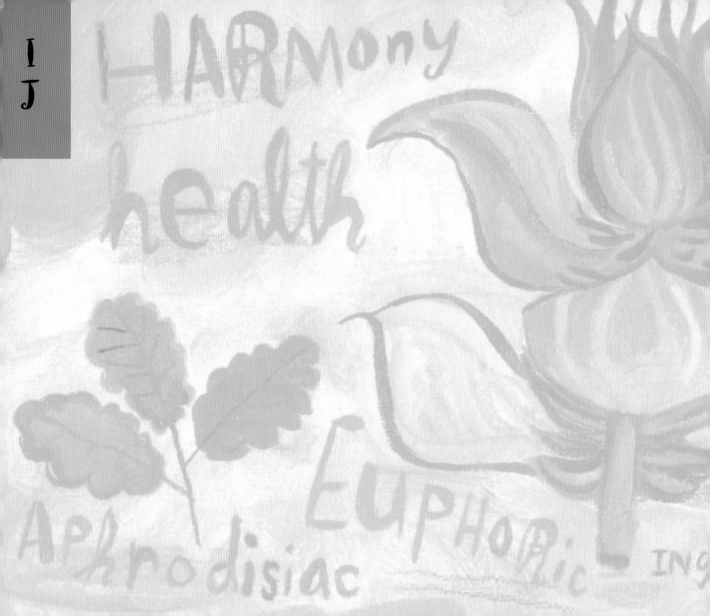

IMMUNE SYSTEM

Cistus, geranium, lavender, lemon*, melaleuca, rosemary (supports immune system), thyme (immunological functions), wild tansy, and white lotus

STIMULATES

Cinnamon*, frankincense*, lavender (for nervous immune system), melaleuca, mountain savory, oregano*; apply to bottoms of feet, along spine, under arms; dilute for massage, and diffuse for 1/2 hour at a time.

BOOSTING IMMUNE DEFENSE

Black cumin
Teas: Gojo berry

IMPETIGO

Boil 4 oz. water, cool, add 5 to 10 drops lavender and wash. You may also use myrrh (cover for an hour). Apply hot compress to site. (Contagious to self and others; treat as soon as noticed.)

IMPOTENCY

Clary sage*, clove*, ginger*, jasmine, nutmeg, rose, sandalwood*, ylang-ylang

INCONTINENCE
(SEE BLADDER)

INDIFFERENCE

Jasmine

INDIGESTION

Ginger, lavender*, peppermint, nutmeg

INFECTION
(SEE ANTI-INFECTIOUS)

Bergamot, cinnamon bark, clove, clary sage*, cypress, jasmine (bacterial infection), juniper, fennel, lavender*, lemongrass, melaleuca (viral), myrrh (fungal infection), oregano, peppermint, ravensara, rosemary* (oral infection), thyme (urinary infection), wild tansy

FUNGICIDAL

Cedarwood

INFECTED WOUNDS

Frankincense, melaleuca, patchouly
To draw out infection: 1 drop thyme; apply
hot compress twice daily. Mix together 3
drops lavender, 2 drops melaleuca, and 2
drops thyme with 1 tsp. pure vegetable oil.
After the infection and pus have been
expelled, apply a little of the mixture twice
daily on infected area.

INFECTIOUS DISEASE

Bergamot, cinnamon bark, clove, ginger,
lemon*, melaleuca, myrtle

BACTERIAL INFECTION

Thyme

VIRAL INFECTION

Hyssop, juniper

INFERIORITY

OVERCOMING

Peppermint

INFERTILITY

(SEE HORMONAL IMBALANCE)

Bergamot, chamomile (Roman), clary sage,
cypress, fennel, geranium, nutmeg, sage,
thyme, yarrow, ylang-ylang.

INFLAMMATION

(SEE ANTI-INFLAMMATORY)

Birch, chamomile, clove, frankincense,
helichrysum, lavender*, myrrh, and spruce

INJURIES

SPORT

Helichrysum

INSECTS

BITES (SEE BITES)

Bergamot
Blend: combine 3 drops chamomile, 4
drops eucalyptus, 10 drops lavender, and 1
drop thyme with 1 Tbl. pure vegetable oil.

INSECTICIDAL

Citronella

REPELLENT

Bergamot

Blend #1: Combine 5 drops lavender, 5 drops lemongrass, 3 drops peppermint, and 1 drop thyme; put on feet or add to cup of water and spray on.

Blend #2: Clove, lemon, and orange

INSOMNIA

Angelica, chamomile (Roman; small amount), clary sage, cypress*, lavender*, lemon*, marjoram*, myrtle* (for hormone-related insomnia), nutmeg (small amount), orange*, ravensara*, rosemary, sandalwood, ylang-ylang*

Combine: 2 drops chamomile, 6 drops geranium, 3 drops lemon, and 4 drops sandalwood. Add 6 drops of mixture in your bath at bedtime and 5 drops with 2 tsps. pure vegetable oil for a massage after bath.

FOR CHILDREN 12 MONTHS TO 5 YEARS

Chamomile (Roman), lavender

5 TO 12 YEARS

Clary sage, geranium, nutmeg, ylang-ylang (infection)

INTESTINAL PROBLEMS

Basil*, bergamot*, ginger, patchouly (aids in the digestion of toxic waste), rosemary, tarragon

ANTISEPTIC

Nutmeg

CRAMPS

Clary sage*

FLORA

Royaldophilus

PARASITES

Clove*, fennel*, lemon*, marjoram*, peppermint, ravensara*

SOOTHE

Spearmint

SPASM

Tarragon*

INVIGORATING

Birch

IN SUMMER

Eucalyptus, peppermint

IONS (IN AIR GIVE ENERGY)

INCREASE NEGATIVE IONS
Bergamot, cedarwood, cypress, grapefruit, orange, patchouly, sandalwood

IRRITABILITY

All single oils *except*: Eucalyptus, pepper, peppermint, and rosemary.

IRRITABLE BOWEL SYNDROME

Peppermint

ITCHING

Lavender, peppermint (ears). Apply on location, too.

JAUNDICE (LIVER DISEASE)

Geranium, lemon, rosemary

JEALOUSY

Bergamot, eucalyptus, frankincense, lemon, marjoram, orange, rose, rosemary, sandalwood, thyme

JET LAG

Eucalyptus, geranium, grapefruit, lavender, lemongrass, peppermint. Apply to temples, thymus, and bottoms of feet.

JOINTS

ACHING
Nutmeg, spruce

DISCOMFORT
Birch

INFLAMED
Chamomile

JOYOUS

Bergamot (turns grief to joy), orange (aromatic)

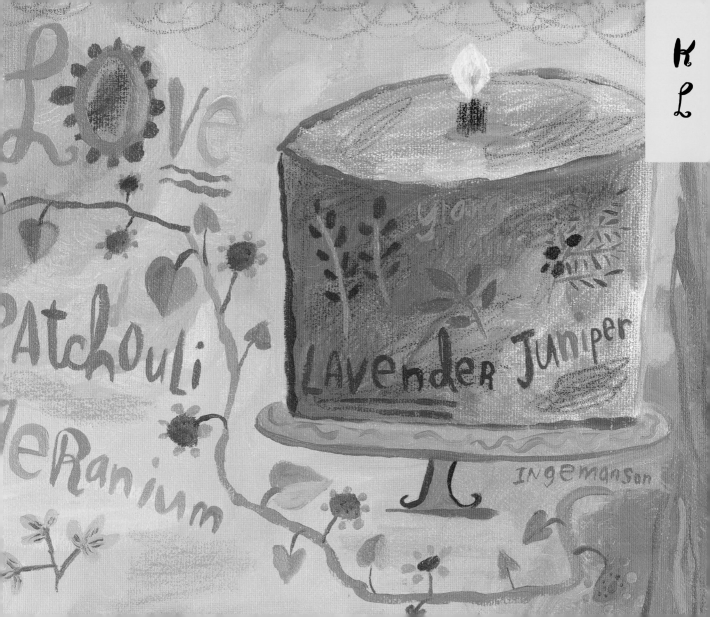

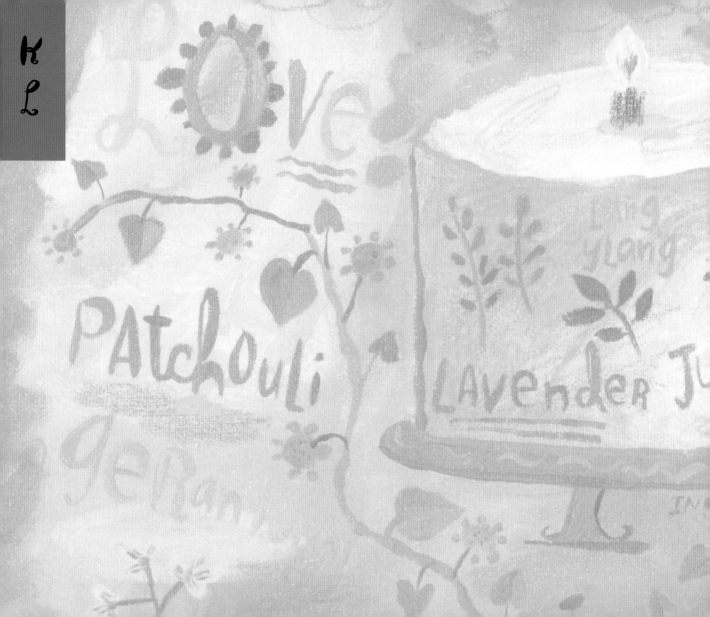

KIDNEYS

Clary sage, geranium, grapefruit, juniper (for better function of kidneys), lemongrass*; apply over kidneys as a hot compress. When kidneys start producing ammonia, it goes to the brain and people can die from it.
Tea: Gojo berry

STONES

Eucalyptus, hyssop, juniper
Apply a hot compress of 10 drops juniper and 10 drops geranium over kidneys once a day.

KNEE CARTILAGE INJURY

Blend 8 drops clove, 12 drops ginger, 10 drops nutmeg, with 2 oz. pure vegetable oil. Massage three times a day. Apply ice for swelling and inflammation. Wrap knee and elevate when sitting. Use the ice method three times a day and alternate with a hot oil compress.

LABOR

(SEE PREGNANCY)
Jasmine (pain), nutmeg (balances hormones during pregnancy, delivery, and after childbirth)

LACTATION

(SEE NURSING)
Fennel*

LARYNGITIS

Jasmine, sandalwood
Diffuse: Frankincense, lavender, sandalwood, thyme

LAXATIVE

Hyssop, jasmine, tangerine

LETHARGY

Jasmine

LICE

Eucalyptus, geranium, lavender, lemon, rosemary; apply to bottoms of feet, rub over scalp three times a day.

LIGAMENTS

Lemongrass

LIPS

Chamomile (German), lavender, lemon, melaleuca

DRY LIPS

Blend 2 to 5 drops geranium with 2 to 5 drops lavender.

LISTLESSNESS

Jasmine

LIVER

Chamomile (Roman), cypress, dill, geranium*(cleanses and detoxifies), grapefruit (liver disorders), helichrysum*, ravensara, sage* (for liver illnesses)
Tea: Gojo berry

CIRRHOSIS

Chamomile, frankincense, geranium, juniper, lavender, myrrh, rosemary, rose

JAUNDICE (LIVER DISEASE)

Geranium*

STIMULANT FOR LIVER CELL FUNCTION

Helichrysum*
Tea: Gojo berry

LONGEVITY

Fennel (aromatic)

LOSS OF LOVED ONE

Basil, cypress (diffuse)

LOSS OF SMELL

Basil

LOVE

Juniper, lavender, ylang-ylang

LUMBAGO

(SEE BACK PAIN)

Sandalwood

LUNGS

(SEE RESPIRATORY SYSTEM)

Eucalyptus, frankincense (stimulates), hyssop (diffuse to clear lungs of mucus), ravensara

PULMONARY

Cypress*, eucalyptus, sage*, sandalwood*

LYMPHATIC SYSTEM

Cypress* (aromatic), sandalwood, tangerine

BALANCE AND LONGEVITY

Blend: Combine 5 drops chamomile, 5 drops lavender, and 5 drops orange in 2 Tbls. pure vegetable oil; massage.

CLEANSING

Lemon

Tea: Gojo berry

DECONGESTANT FOR

Cypress*, grapefruit*, myrtle

DRAINAGE OF

Helichrysum*, lemongrass*

ELIMINATES WASTE THROUGH

Lavender*

INCREASE FUNCTION OF

Lemon

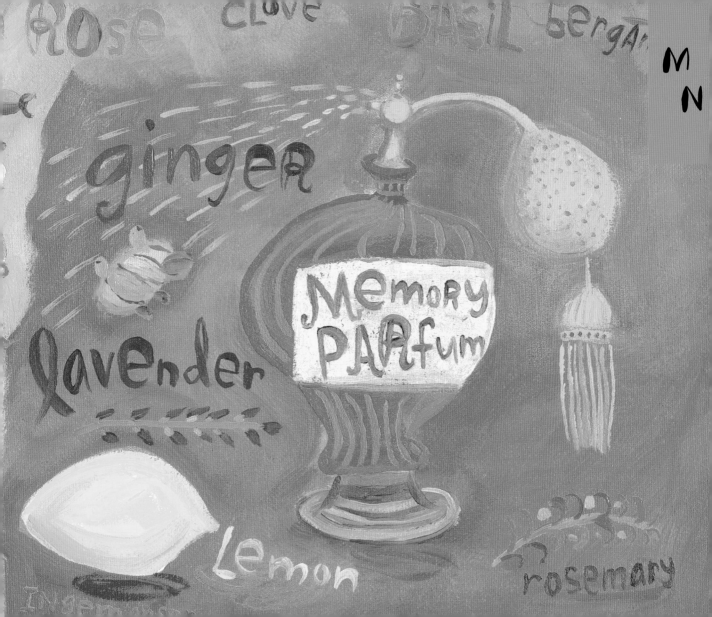

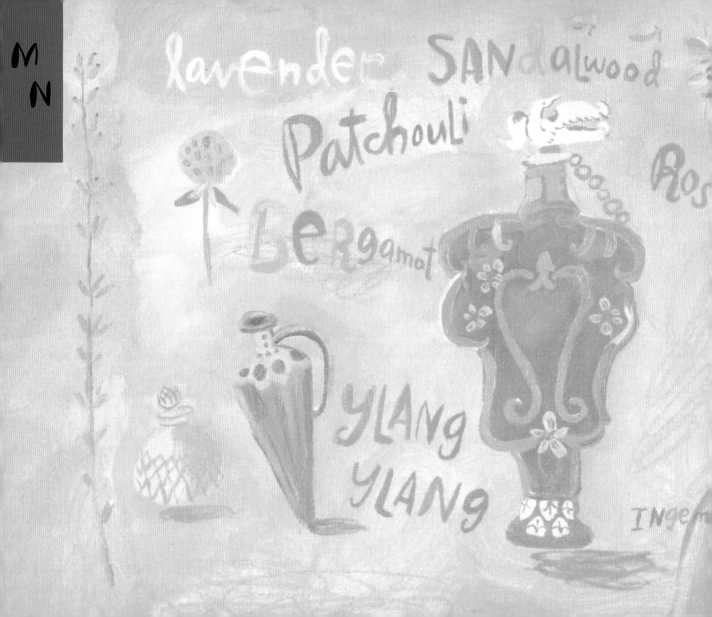

MALARIA

Lemon with honey in water to prevent.

MALE GENITAL AREA

INFECTION

Eucalyptus, lavender, melaleuca, oregano, patchouly

INFLAMMATION

Chamomile, hyssop, lavender

SWELLING

Cypress, eucalyptus, hyssop, juniper, lavender, rosemary

INFERTILITY

Basil, cedarwood, clary sage, sage, thyme

JOCK ITCH

Cypress, lavender, melaleuca, or patchouly. Put 2 drops of any of these oils in 1 tsp. pure vegetable oil and apply to area morning and night; or put 2 drops of any of these oils in a small bowl of water and wash and dry area well.

MASSAGE

Blend (relaxing massage): 5 drops chamomile, 5 drops lavender, 5 drops orange with 2 Tbls. pure vegetable oil.

MEASLES

(SEE CHILDHOOD DISEASES)

Eucalyptus

MEDITATION

Chamomile, myrrh (aromatic), sandalwood

MELANOMA

(SEE CANCER)

OF SKIN

Frankincense and lavender

MEMORY

Basil (for poor memory), bergamot, clove (memory deficiency), ginger, grapefruit, lavender, lemon (improves), rose, rosemary. Wear as a perfume, apply to temples, and diffuse.

IMPROVE

Clary sage (aromatic), clove
Blend: 5 drops basil, 2 drops peppermint, 10 drops rosemary, and 1 oz. pure vegetable oil.

RELEASE NEGATIVE

Geranium (aromatic)

STIMULATE

Rosemary (aromatic)
Blend: 2 drops blue tansy, 2 drops chamomile, 3 drops geranium, 4 drops lavender, 3 drops rosemary, 3 drops rosewood, 1 drop spearmint, 2 drops tangerine, and 1 oz. pure vegetable oil. Apply to back of neck, wrist, and heart.

MENOPAUSE

(SEE HORMONAL IMBALANCE)

Basil, bergamot, chamomile, clary sage, cypress*, fennel*, geranium, jasmine, lavender*, nutmeg (balances hormones), sage*, thyme. Apply oil(s) to feet, ankles, lower back, groin, and pelvis.

PREMENOPAUSE

Clary sage*, fennel*, lavender*, nutmeg (balances hormones), orange*, tarragon*

MENSTRUAL

(SEE HORMONAL IMBALANCE)

Basil* (scanty periods)

CRAMPS

Clary sage*, cypress* (pain)

PAINFUL PERIODS

Chamomile (Roman), cypress, geranium, jasmine, lavender, nutmeg (balances hormones), peppermint, sage, tarragon, thyme

PREMENSTRUAL SYNDROME (PMS)

Grapefruit

PROMOTE

Sage

REGULATE

Peppermint*, rosemary*, sage*

MENTAL

Oregano (mental diseases), sage (strain, aromatic)

ACCURACY

Peppermint

FATIGUE

Basil*, rosemary*, sage (diffuse), ylang-ylang*

METABOLISM

BALANCE

Clove (aromatic), oregano, spearmint

INCREASE (OVERALL)

Spearmint

LIPID

Hyssop (regulates)

STRENGTHENING (VITAL CENTERS)

Sage

METAL

Helichrysum

PULL OUT

Blend: Combine 10 drops cypress, 10 drops juniper, 10 drops lemongrass with 1 oz. pure vegetable oil and massage body.

MIGRAINE HEADACHES

(SEE HEADACHES)

Basil*, chamomile (German), eucalyptus*, grapefruit, lavender, marjoram*, peppermint*, spearmint

MIND

OPEN

Basil (absentminded)

MISCARRIAGE

(SEE PREGNANCY)

MOLES

Frankincense, geranium, lavender

MOOD SWINGS

(SEE HORMONAL IMBALANCE)

Bergamot, clary sage, fennel, geranium,
jasmine, juniper, lavender, lemon,
peppermint, rose, rosemary, sage,
sandalwood, spruce, yarrow, ylang-ylang

MORNING SICKNESS

(SEE PREGNANCY)

MOTION SICKNESS

Ginger, nutmeg, peppermint, spearmint;
apply to feet, temples, and wrists.

MOTIVATION

TO MOVE FORWARD

Myrrh

MUCUS

(SEE ANTICATARRHAL)

Cypress*, helichrysum (discharge), and/or
rosemary*

MULTIPLE SCLEROSIS (MS)

Cypress, geranium, juniper, oregano,
peppermint, rosemary, and thyme. Do
raindrop therapy.
Blend: Combine 6 drops juniper, 4 drops
sandalwood, 2 drops peppermint, 12 drops
geranium; mix and massage into neck,
spine, and bottoms of feet.

MUMPS

(SEE CHILDHOOD DISEASES)

Lavender, melaleuca

MUSCLES

ACHES AND PAINS

Birch*, ginger, nutmeg, rosemary

ANTI-INFLAMMATORY

Peppermint

CRAMPS

Chamomile, clary sage, cypress, lavender (aromatic), marjoram, rosemary

FATIGUE

Cypress, grapefruit, marjoram, ravensara, rosemary, thyme

SHOULDERS

Helichrysum, spruce

SPASMS

Basil, clary sage, lavender, jasmine, marjoram, chamomile (Roman)

STIFFNESS

Basil, bergamot, geranium, lavender, lemon, marjoram, nutmeg, orange, rosemary, thyme

TENSION

Chamomile (blue)

TORN MUSCLES

Helichrysum and spruce take pain away (use hot packs).

RELAXING OILS

Basil, eucalyptus, ginger, rosemary

STIMULATING OILS

Geranium, lavender, lemon, orange

MUSCULAR DYSTROPHY

Basil, eucalyptus, geranium, ginger, lavender, lemon, orange, rosemary

NAILS

Eucalyptus, grapefruit, lavender, lemon, melaleuca, myrrh, oregano, patchouly, peppermint, ravensara, rosemary, thyme

NASAL

(SEE NOSE)

NAUSEA

Clove, ginger, juniper, lavender*, nutmeg, peppermint* (aromatic), rosewood, spearmint, tarragon; apply behind ears. Blend: Combine 2 drops lavender, 2 drops spearmint, and 2 drops of another oil for your type of nausea; mix together and put a little on a cotton ball and inhale three times a day or diffuse.

NECK

Basil, clary sage, geranium, lemon, lemongrass, orange, helichrysum; apply oils to base of big toe.

NEGATIVITY

Sandalwood (Removes negative programming from the cells.)

DROWNING IN OWN

Grapefruit (aromatic)

NERVOUS SYSTEM

Basil* (stimulant and for nervous breakdown), bergamot, cedarwood (nervous tension), chamomile (Roman), cinnamon bark, frankincense, geranium (regenerates nerves), jasmine (nervous exhaustion), juniper (better nerve function), lavender, lemon, lemongrass (for nerve damage; activates), marjoram (soothing), nutmeg (supports), orange, palmarosa (supports), pepper (stimulant), peppermint (soothes and strengthens), ravensara*, rosemary, sage*, sandalwood, spearmint, spruce (fatigue)

NERVOUSNESS

Cypress, orange, tangerine

PARASYMPATHETIC NERVES *(SEE PARASYMPATHETIC NERVES)*

Marjoram* (increases tone of)

VIRUS OF NERVES

Clove and frankincense

NEURALGIA

(SEVERE PAIN ALONG NERVE)

Cedarwood, chamomile, eucalyptus, helichrysum, juniper, lavender, marjoram*, nutmeg

NEURITIS

Cedarwood, chamomile, eucalyptus, juniper, lavender

NEUROMUSCULAR

Tarragon

NEUROPATHY

Cedarwood, chamomile, eucalyptus, juniper, lavender

NEUROTONIC

Melaleuca, thyme

NIGHT SWEATS

(SEE HOT FLASHES AND HORMONAL IMBALANCE)
Sage*

NOSE

Melaleuca, rosemary

BLEEDING

Cypress, frankincense, lavender, lemon
Blend: Combine 2 drops cypress, 1 drop helichrysum, and 2 drops lemon in 8 oz. ice water; soak cloth and apply to nose and back of neck.

NASAL MUCUS MEMBRANE

Eucalyptus may help reduce inflammation.

NASAL NASOPHARYNX

Eucalyptus

POLYPS IN NOSE

Basil

NURSING

Clary sage (brings in milk production), fennel* (increases milk production), geranium
Blend: Combine 7 to 15 drops fennel, 7 to 15 drops geranium, or 5 to 10 drops clary sage; use one oil in 2 Tbls. pure vegetable oil.

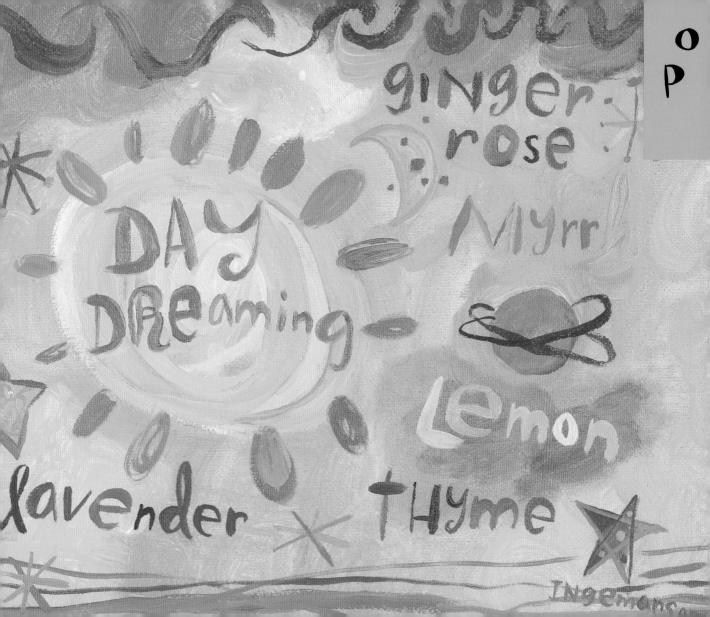

OBESITY

(SEE WEIGHT)

Fennel, grapefruit, juniper, orange, rosemary, tangerine

REDUCE

Orange, tangerine

OBSESSIVENESS

Clary sage, cypress, geranium, helichrysum, lavender, marjoram, rose, sandalwood, ylang-ylang

ODORS

Bergamot, lavender

CONTROLLING

Cedarwood

OPENING (TO RECEIVE)

Fir (aromatic)

ORAL INFECTIONS

Rosewood*

OSTEOPOROSIS

(SEE HORMONAL IMBALANCE)

Birch, chamomile (Roman and German), clove, fennel, fir, geranium, ginger, hyssop, lemon, nutmeg, oregano, peppermint, pine, rosemary, spruce, and thyme

OVARIES

(SEE HORMONAL IMBALANCE)

Geranium, myrtle*, and/or rosemary* (regulates)

OVERCOME AND RELEASE UNPLEASANT, DIFFICULT ISSUES

Chamomile

OVEREATING
(SEE EATING DISORDERS)

OVERWEIGHT
(SEE OBESITY AND WEIGHT)

OXYGEN

All essential oils increase the ability of the body to take oxygen to the cells and to push toxins out. The oils pick up more oxygen and take it to the site of discomfort.

OXYGENATING
Fennel, fir, oregano

PAIN

Birch, clove*, eucalyptus, helichrysum, jasmine (relieves), spruce (reduces pain from torn muscles), rosemary (muscle), tarragon* (rheumatic)

GROWING PAINS
Massage with birch, cypress, and peppermint.

REDUCING
Helichrysum*, marjoram*

PAINTING

Add one 15 ml. bottle of your favorite blend of oil to any five-gallon bucket of paint. Stir vigorously, mixing well, and then either spray paint or paint by hand. This should eliminate the paint fumes and after-smell.

PALPITATIONS
(SEE HEART)

PANCREAS

Coriander, cypress* (for insufficiencies), dill

STIMULANT FOR
Helichrysum*

SUPPORT
Cinnamon, fennel, and geranium

PANCREATITIS

WEAKNESS
Lemon, marjoram

PANIC

Bergamot, birch, chamomile (Roman), fir, frankincense, lavender, marjoram, myrrh, rosemary, sandalwood, spruce, thyme, ylang-ylang

PARALYSIS

Cypress, geranium, helichrysum, juniper, peppermint
Blend: Combine 6 drops cypress, 15 drops geranium, 10 drops helichrysum, 5 drops juniper, 2 drops peppermint, and pure vegetable oil. May rejuvenate nerve damage up to 60 percent. Put on location and feet.

PARASITES

(SEE ANTIPARASITIC)

Clove, fennel*, hyssop, melaleuca, mountain savory, oregano*, tangerine, tarragon*, thyme; apply oil on stomach and feet to help pass parasites.

ANTIPARASITIC

Nutmeg*

INTESTINAL

Lemon*, marjoram*, ravensara*

PARASYMPATHETIC NERVOUS SYSTEM

Lemongrass* (regulates), marjoram* (increases tone of)

PARKINSON'S DISEASE

Basil, bergamot, cypress (circulation), frankincense, geranium, helichrysum, juniper, lavender, lemon, marjoram, nutmeg, orange, peppermint, rosemary, sandalwood, thyme

PEACE

Juniper (aromatic), lavender (aromatic), marjoram, ylang-ylang

FINDING

Tangerine (aromatic)

PROMOTING

Chamomile

Pelvic Pain Syndrome

Bergamot, clove, geranium, ginger, nutmeg, thyme

Personal Growth

ELIMINATING BLOCKS

Helichrysum, frankincense

Pest Troubles

(SEE INSECTS)

Ravensara*

pH Balance

A state where the pH is alkaline inside the blood, and acid outside the blood. When not balanced, the body creates a climate for illness. Cancer and candida need an acid condition to survive. The more acidic, the less synergistic the oils will be to the body. In acidic conditions, the oils take longer to work and don't last as long. The body can only heal in an alkaline state. Lemon converts to alkaline the moment it goes in the mouth. Some types of water may cause acid condition; add lemon to the water.

Phlebitis

Chamomile (Roman), cypress, geranium, grapefruit, helichrysum* (prevents), lavender*; massage toward heart and wear support hose until healed, possibly 2 to 3 months. Do raindrop therapy on leg.

Pimples

Clary sage

Pineal Gland

OPENS

Cedarwood, sandalwood (increases oxygen), spruce

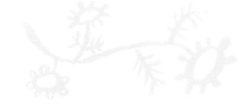

PITUITARY

Sandalwood increases oxygen around the pituitary gland.

BALANCES

Geranium, ylang-ylang; apply to forehead and back of neck.

PLAGUE

Clove*

PLEURISY

Cypress*

PMS (PREMENSTRUAL SYNDROME)

(SEE HORMONAL IMBALANCE)

Bergamot, chamomile (Roman), clary sage*, fennel, geranium, grapefruit, jasmine, lavender (aromatic), nutmeg

APATHETIC, TIRED, LISTLESS

Bergamot, chamomile (Roman), fennel, geranium, grapefruit

IRRITABLE, DISAGREEABLE

Bergamot, chamomile (Roman), clary sage, nutmeg

VIOLENT, AGGRESSIVE

Bergamot, geranium, nutmeg

WEEPING, DEPRESSION

Bergamot, clary sage, geranium, nutmeg

PNEUMONIA

(SEE RESPIRATORY SYSTEM)

Eucalyptus, frankincense, lavender, lemon, melaleuca, oregano, ravensara, and thyme are good to use as compresses.

POISON OAK/IVY

Chamomile (Roman), lavender

POLLUTION

(SEE PURIFICATION)

AIR

Lemon, peppermint

WATER

Lemon, peppermint

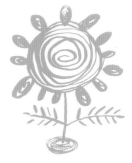

PREGNANCY

Chamomile (Roman), geranium, grapefruit, jasmine, lavender, tangerine, ylang-ylang

DELIVERY

Clary sage, lavender (stimulates circulation, calming, antibiotic, anti-inflammatory, antiseptic), nutmeg (balances hormones, calms the central nervous system, alleviates anxiety, increases circulation, and good for blood supply)

EARLY LABOR

Lavender

ENERGY

Put equal portions of chamomile (Roman), geranium, and lavender in pure vegetable oil.

LABOR

Geranium, lavender

MISCARRIAGE (AFTER)

Chamomile (Roman), frankincense, geranium, grapefruit

MORNING SICKNESS

Ginger, nutmeg, peppermint (over stomach, behind ears), or spearmint (4 to 6 drops in bowl of boiled and cooled water and place on floor beside the bed overnight to keep stomach calm)

POSTPARTUM (BABY BLUES)

(SEE FEMALE PROBLEMS)

Bergamot, clary sage, fennel, frankincense, geranium, grapefruit, lavender, myrrh, nutmeg, and patchouly

UTERUS

Tone with 1 to 3 drops of clary sage around ankles.
Fennel, sage

TRANSITION

Basil

PRIDE

Peppermint (dispels)

PROSPERITY

Bergamot, cinnamon bark (aromatic), cypress*

PROSTATE

DECONGEST

Cypress, myrrh, myrtle*, sage, spruce*;
apply oils to inside ankle and heel.
Blend: Combine 10 drops frankincense and
10 drops lavender with 2 tsps. pure
vegetable oil; insert blend into rectum with
bulb syringe and retain throughout night.

INFLAMED

Cypress, lavender, thyme

PROSTATE CANCER

(SEE CANCER)

PROTECTION

FROM NEGATIVE INFLUENCE

Clove (aromatic), cypress, fennel
(protection from psychic attack), fir
(aromatic), frankincense

PSORIASIS

Bergamot, cedarwood, chamomile,
helichrysum*, lavender, thyme
Blend 2 to 3 drops of chamomile and
lavender for use as ointment for pH
balance.

PSYCHIC

Lemongrass (aromatic)

AWARENESS

Cinnamon bark (aromatic)

PULMONARY

(SEE LUNGS)

PURIFICATION

Cedarwood, eucalyptus (aromatic), fennel
(aromatic), lemon (aromatic), lemongrass
(aromatic), melaleuca (aromatic), orange
(aromatic), sage

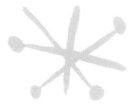

DISHES

Add 2 drops of lemon in dishwater for sparkling dishes and a great-smelling kitchen.

WATER

Lemon*, peppermint

CLOTHING

Adding oils to washer or dryer increases antibacterial and hygiene, and give clothes a refreshing, clean smell.

FURNITURE

A few drops of fir, lemon, or spruce oil on a dust cloth, or 10 drops in a spray bottle, work well for polishing, cleaning, and disinfecting furniture, kitchens, and bathrooms. Use lemon oil for dissolving gum and grease.

PUS

(SEE INFECTION AND ANTI-INFECTIOUS)

Melaleuca is useful in healing pus-filled wounds.

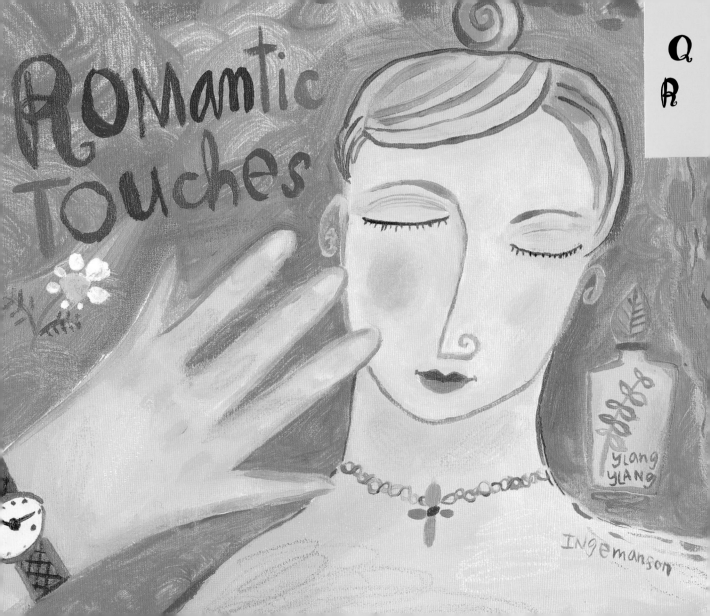

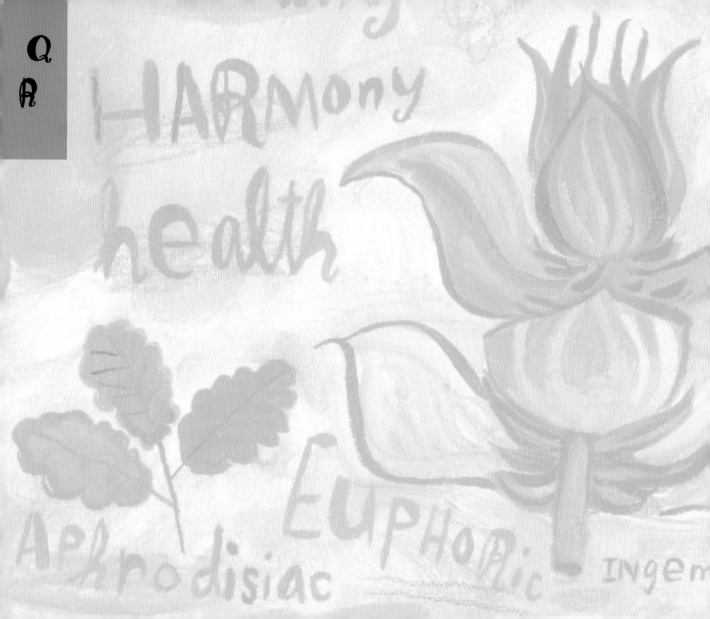

RADIATION

Melaleuca; may apply on location, bottoms of feet, kidneys, thyroid, and diffuse.

WEEPING WOUNDS FROM

Melaleuca, oregano, thyme

RASHES

Chamomile, lavender, melaleuca*, palmarosa

RAYNAUD'S DISEASE

FEEL COLD; HANDS AND FEET TURN BLUE

Clove, fennel, geranium, lavender, nutmeg, rosemary

REGENERATING

Helichrysum, lavender

RELATIONSHIPS

ENHANCING

Ylang-ylang

ENDING RELATIONSHIPS

Basil

RELAXATION

Clary sage, frankincense, geranium, jasmine, sandalwood, ylang-ylang
Blend: Combine 1 drop bergamot, 2 drops lavender, 2 drops marjoram, and 4 drops rosewood.

RESENTMENT

Jasmine, rose, tansy

RESPIRATORY SYSTEM

Basil (restorative), clary sage (strengthens), clove, eucalyptus* (general stimulant and strengthens), fennel (stimulant), fir (opens respiratory track, increases oxygenation, decongests and balances), frankincense, helichrysum (relieves), lemon, marjoram

(calming), melaleuca, myrtle*, oregano (antiseptic), peppermint (aid), ravensara, spearmint*, spruce
Blend: Combine 3 drops birch, 8 drops eucalyptus, 6 drops fir, 6 drops frankincense, 1 drop peppermint, 10 drops ravensara, and 1 oz. pure vegetable oil.
Blend: Combine 3 drops birch, 8 drops eucalyptus, 6 drops fir, 6 drops frankincense, 1 drop peppermint, 10 drops ravensara, and 1 oz. pure vegetable oil.
Blend: Combine 3 drops chamomile (blue), 10 drops fir, and 6 drops lemon.
Blend: Combine 5 drops eucalyptus, 8 drops frankincense, 6 drops lemon, and 1 oz. pure vegetable oil. Rub on chest and neat on bottoms of feet under toes. Apply a hot compress to chest.

RESTLESSNESS

Angelica, basil, bergamot, cedarwood, frankincense, geranium, lavender, orange, rose, rosewood, spruce, valor, ylang-ylang

RHEUMATIC FEVER

PAIN OF
Ginger, tarragon*

RHEUMATISM

(RHEUMATOID ARTHRITIS)
Birch*, chamomile, cinnamon bark, cypress*, eucalyptus, fir, geranium, hyssop, juniper, lavender, lemon*, marjoram*, nutmeg*, pepper (black), rosemary, spruce*, tarragon, thyme
CHRONIC
Oregano*
PAIN
Ginger*

RHINITIS (INFLAMMATION OF NASAL MUCUS MEMBRANE)
Basil

RHINOPHARYNGITIS

Ravensara

RINGWORM

Geranium, lavender, melaleuca, myrrh,
peppermint, rosemary, thyme
Blend #1: Combine 2 drops lavender, 2
drops melaleuca, and 2 drops thyme.
Blend #2: Combine 3 drops melaleuca, 2
drops peppermint, and 3 drops spearmint.
Apply 1 to 2 drops of blend on ringworm
three times a day for 10 days. Then mix 30
drops of melaleuca with 2 Tbls. pure
vegetable oil and use daily until ringworm
is gone.

ROMANTIC TOUCHES

Jasmine, patchouly, ylang-ylang; use in
small amounts.

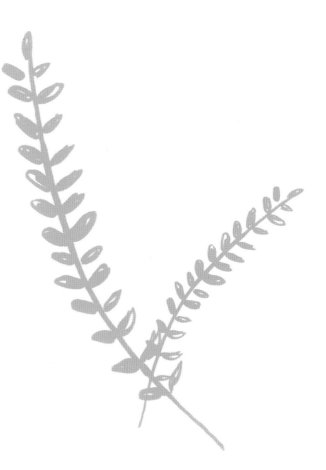

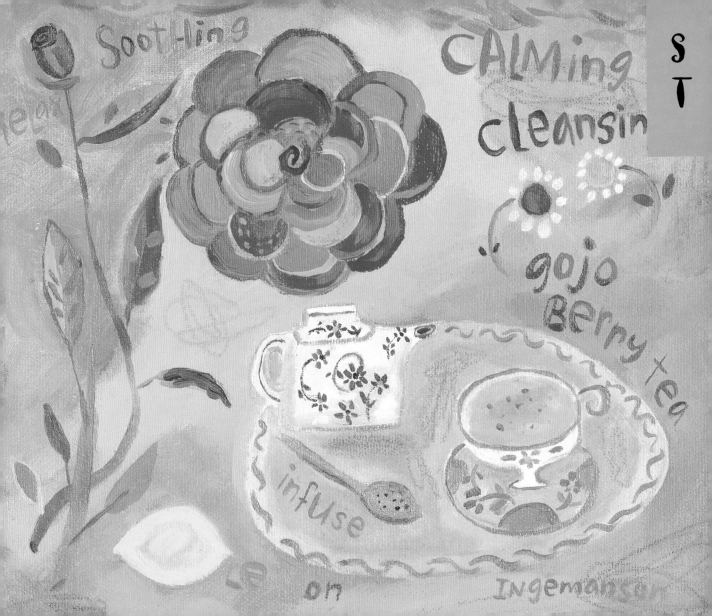

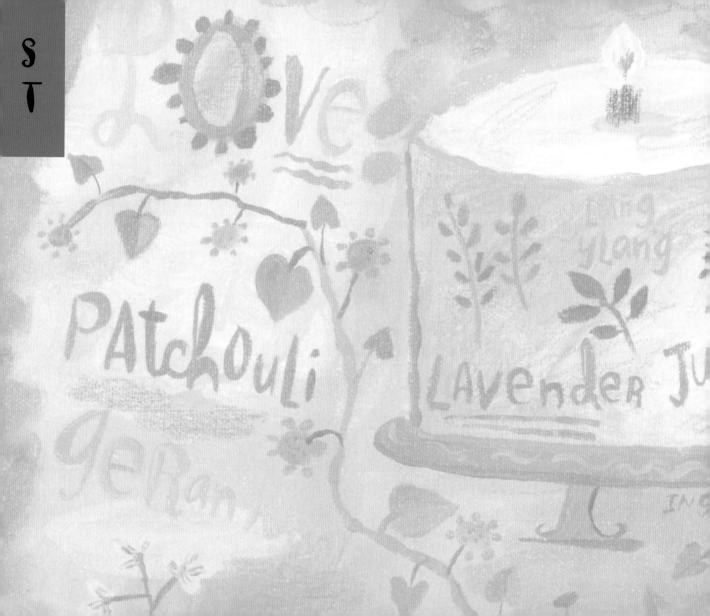

SADNESS

Orange (overcome)

SCABIES

Bergamot

SCARRING

Frankincense (prevents), helichrysum, hyssop (prevents), lavender (burns), rose (prevents)
Blend #1: Combine equal parts helichrysum and lavender mixed with liquid lecithin.
Blend #2: Combine 3 drops rosemary, 15 drops rosewood, and 1 3/4 oz. hazelnut oil.
Blend #3: Combine 6 drops lavender, 3 drops patchouly, 4 drops rosewood, and vitamin E oil.

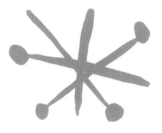

SCIATICA

Fir, helichrysum*, hyssop, peppermint, sandalwood, spruce (alleviates pain), tarragon*, thyme*; apply a cold press and lightly massage with chamomile, lavender, or birch.

SCOLIOSIS

Do raindrop therapy.
Blend: Combine 8 drops basil, 12 drops birch, 5 drops cypress, 10 drops marjoram, and 2 drops peppermint.

SCRAPES

Lavender, ravensara

SCURVY

Ginger. Apply to kidneys, liver, and feet.

SECURITY

CREATING
Chamomile

FEELING OF
Cypress (aromatic)

IN THE HOME
Bergamot

SELF-SECURE
Oregano

SEDATIVE

Angelica, coriander, jasmine, lavender, lemongrass, marjoram*, orange, tangerine

SELF-HYPNOSIS

Clary sage, geranium, patchouly

SENSORY SYSTEM (SENSES)

Birch

SEX STIMULANT

Cinnamon (general), ginger, rose, ylang-ylang* (sex-drive problems)

AROUSE DESIRE
Clary sage

FRIGIDITY *(SEE FRIGIDITY)*
Nutmeg (overcome)

INFLUENCES
Patchouly (aromatic)

SHINGLES (INTERNAL NERVE VIRUS)

Geranium, melaleuca (Need to cleanse the liver.)

HERPES ZOSTER
Bergamot, chamomile, eucalyptus, geranium, lavender, melaleuca

SHOCK
(SEE FAINTING)
Basil, chamomile (Roman), helichrysum, melaleuca, myrrh, peppermint*, rosemary, ylang-ylang

SINUS

Cedarwood, eucalyptus, helichrysum*, myrtle, rosemary*

SINUSITIS

(SEE RESPIRATORY SYSTEM)

Eucalyptus*, fir, ginger, myrtle, ravensara

SKIN

(SEE ACNE, ALLERGIES, DERMATITIS, ECZEMA, FACIAL OILS, AND PSORIASIS)

Cedarwood, Roman and blue chamomile (inflamed skin), cypress, frankincense, geranium, helichrysum, jasmine (irritated skin), juniper, lavender, lemon, marjoram, melaleuca (healing), myrrh (chapped and cracked), myrtle* (antiseptic), orange, palmarosa (rashes, scaly and flaky skin), peppermint (itching), rosemary, rosewood (elasticity and candida), sage, sandalwood (regenerates), and ylang-ylang

DISEASE

Rose

DRY

Chamomile, davana (dry and chapped), geranium, jasmine, lavender, lemon, patchouly, rosewood*, sandalwood

OILY

Bergamot, clary sage, cypress, jasmine, lavender, lemon, nutmeg, orange, ylang-ylang

SENSITIVE

Chamomile (German), geranium, jasmine, lavender

SLEEP

Chamomile (aromatic), lavender (on spine), marjoram (aromatic)

ANIMALS

Oils can be used on the paws to help animals relax and sleep when in pain.

RESTFUL

Combine 1/4 cup bath salts, 10 drops geranium or lavender in bath and soak.

RESTLESS

Lavender

SLEEPING SICKNESS

Geranium, juniper, peppermint

SLIMMING AND TONING OILS

Basil, grapefruit, lavender, lemongrass, orange, rosemary, sage, thyme

SMELL

LOSS OF SENSE

Basil helps when due to chronic nasal catarrh.

SOOTHING

Chamomile, myrrh

SORES

Melaleuca

SORE THROAT

(SEE THROAT)

SPASMS

Basil, chamomile (Roman), cypress*, lavender* (antispasmodic), marjoram (relieves), oregano, peppermint, and thyme

SPASTICITY

Cypress, ginger, juniper, lavender, lemon, rosemary, sandalwood

SPINA BIFIDA (CONGENITAL DEFECT OF BACKBONE)

Work on nervous system with chamomile, eucalyptus, lavender, lemon, nutmeg, orange, rosemary. Apply oil(s) to bottoms of feet, along spine, forehead, back of neck, and diffuse. Do raindrop therapy.

SPINE

CALCIFIED

Geranium, rosemary

STIFFNESS

Marjoram; do raindrop therapy.

SPIRITUAL

AWARENESS

Cedarwood, juniper, myrrh, spruce

BALANCING SPIRITUAL AWARENESS

Spruce

INCREASE

Frankincense (opening and enhancing spiritual receptivity; aromatic), cedarwood (enhances)

MEDITATION

Frankincense

PURITY OF SPIRIT

Myrrh

SPORTS

INJURIES

Helichrysum

TRACK COMPETITION

Blend: Combine 5 drops basil, 5 drops bergamot, and 2 tsps. pure vegetable oil.

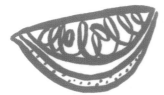

SPRAINS

Ginger, jasmine, lavender, marjoram*, rose, sage. Make a cold compress with chamomile, eucalyptus, lavender, or rosemary.

SPURS (BONE)

(SEE BONES)

Lavender

STAINS

Lemon (removes)

STAPH INFECTION

Pepper or peppermint will make it more painful. Use oregano and hyssop and oregano and thyme to relieve the pain. Helichrysum, lavender

STERILITY

Clary sage, geranium*

STIMULATING

Ginger, grapefruit, orange, peppermint*, rose, sage*

STINGS

(SEE BITES)

STOMACH

Basil*, ginger

ACHE

Eucalyptus, geranium, lavender, peppermint, or rosemary

ACID

Peppermint (Put drop on finger and place on tongue.)

CRAMPS

Helichrysum*, lavender*, thyme* (general tonic for)

TONIC

Tangerine

STRENGTH

Chamomile (strengthens positive imprinting in DNA), cypress (aromatic), oregano, patchouly, peppermint*

STREP THROAT

(SEE THROAT)

STRESS

Basil, bergamot, chamomile (Roman—relieves stress), clary sage, cypress, frankincense, geranium, grapefruit, lavender (aromatic), marjoram, rosewood, spruce, tangerine, and ylang-ylang

CHEMICAL

Clary sage, geranium, grapefruit, lavender, lemon, patchouly, rosemary

EMOTIONAL

Bergamot, geranium, and sandalwood (layer on navel and chest)

ENVIRONMENTAL

Basil, bergamot, cedarwood, chamomile (Roman), cypress, geranium

MENTAL

Basil, bergamot, geranium, grapefruit, lavender, patchouly, sandalwood

PERFORMANCE

Bergamot, ginger, grapefruit, rosemary

PHYSICAL

Bergamot, chamomile (Roman), fennel, geranium, lavender, marjoram, rosemary, thyme

RELATIONSHIP *(SEE SEX STIMULANT)*

TIREDNESS, IRRITABILITY OR INSOMNIA

Blend: Combine 15 drops clary sage, 10 drops lemon, 5 drops lavender, and 1 oz. pure vegetable oil

STRETCH MARKS

Lavender*, myrrh*
Blend #1: Combine 3 drops rosemary, 15 drops rosewood, and 1 3/4 oz. hazelnut oil.
Blend #2: Combine 6 drops lavender, 4 drops rosewood, 3 drops patchouly, and vitamin E oil.

STROKE

HEAT

Lavender or peppermint (rub on neck and forehead)

MUSCULAR PARALYSIS

Lavender
Blend: Combine equal parts of basil, lavender, and rosemary. Rub spinal column and paralyzed area.

STRUCTURAL ALIGNMENT

Basil, birch, cypress, peppermint. Do raindrop therapy.

SUBCONSCIOUS

Helichrysum (uplifts when diffused)

SUICIDE

(SEE DEPRESSION AND EMOTIONS)

SUNBURN

Melaleuca*; spray or rub with chamomile and lavender.

PREVENT BLISTERING

Apply 2 to 3 drops of lavender.

SUNSCREEN

Helichrysum*

SUPPORTIVE

Myrrh

SWELLING

Lemongrass, tangerine

TACHYCARDIA

Lavender, orange, ylang-ylang. Apply to heart area.

TALKATIVE

Cypress (overtalkative)

TASTE

Helichrysum (1 drop on tongue)

TEETH

GUM SURGERY

Helichrysum every 15 minutes for pain.

TEETHING PAIN

Chamomile

TOOTHACHE

Chamomile, clove*; apply on location and along jawbone.

TOOTHPASTE

Combine 4 tsps. green or white clay, 1 tsp. salt, 1 to 2 drops peppermint, 1 to 2 drops lemon; mix clockwise.

TEMPERATURE

(SEE FEVER OR THYROID)

TENDINITIS

Basil, birch, cypress, lavender, ginger, peppermint, and rosemary. Do raindrop therapy.

PAIN RELIEF

Birch and peppermint

TENNIS ELBOW

Combine 10 drops eucalyptus, 10 drops peppermint, 10 drops rosemary, and 1 Tbl. pure vegetable oil; mix, apply, then apply ice pack.

TENSION

Bergamot, cedarwood*, frankincense, lavender

RELIEVE

Chamomile, grapefruit

TESTICLES

Rosemary*

THROAT

Cypress*

DRY

Grapefruit, lemon

INFECTION IN

Clary sage, lemon*, peppermint

LARYNGITIS (SEE LARYNGITIS)

SORE

Rub one of the following on throat: Bergamot, geranium, ginger, melaleuca*, myrrh, sandalwood. Inhalations with clary sage, eucalyptus, lavender, sandalwood, thyme.

STREP

Geranium, ginger

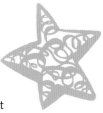

THRUSH

Bergamot, eucalyptus, lavender*, marjoram, rose, thyme

VAGINAL

Geranium, melaleuca*, myrrh*, patchouly, rosemary

THYMUS
Ravensara*

STIMULATES
Spruce*

THYROID

DISFUNCTION
Clove

NORMALIZE HORMONAL IMBALANCE OF
Myrtle

HYPERTHYROID
Myrrh*, myrtle, spruce*

HYPOTHYROID
Myrrh

SUPPORTS
Myrtle (Rub on hands and feet.)

TINNITUS
Juniper, helichrysum; apply to mastoid bone behind ear.

TIRED
(SEE FATIGUE)

TISSUE
Basil, chamomile, lavender, lemongrass, marjoram

BONE AND JOINT REGENERATION
Blend: Combine 5 drops birch, 2 drops chamomile (blue), 1 drop blue tansy, 7 drops fir, 5 drops helichrysum, 5 drops hyssop, 4 drops lemongrass, 8 drops sandalwood, 8 drops spruce, and 1 oz. pure vegetable oil.

CLEANSE TOXINS
Fennel

REPAIR
Helichrysum (for scar tissue; reduces tissue pain), hyssop (scars), lemongrass (repairs connective tissue), orange, rosewood

REGENERATE
Geranium, helichrysum, lemongrass, patchouly*

TONIC

Mountain savory (general tonic for the whole body)

TONSILLITIS

Chamomile (Roman), ginger*, lavender, lemon (gargle), melaleuca*; apply on throat and lungs.

TOOTHACHE

(SEE TEETH)

TOXINS

Fennel, fir, patchouly (digests toxic wastes)

TRANSITION IN LIFE

Basil, cypress

TUBERCULOSIS (TB)

Cedarwood*, cypress*, eucalyptus*, lemon, myrtle*, oregano* (pulmonary), peppermint, sandalwood, thyme*, rose, rosemary

TUMORS

ANTITUMORAL
Clove, frankincense*

TYPHOID

Cinnamon*

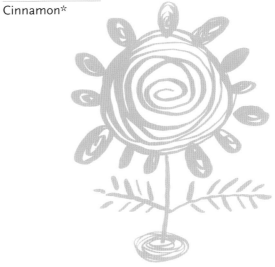

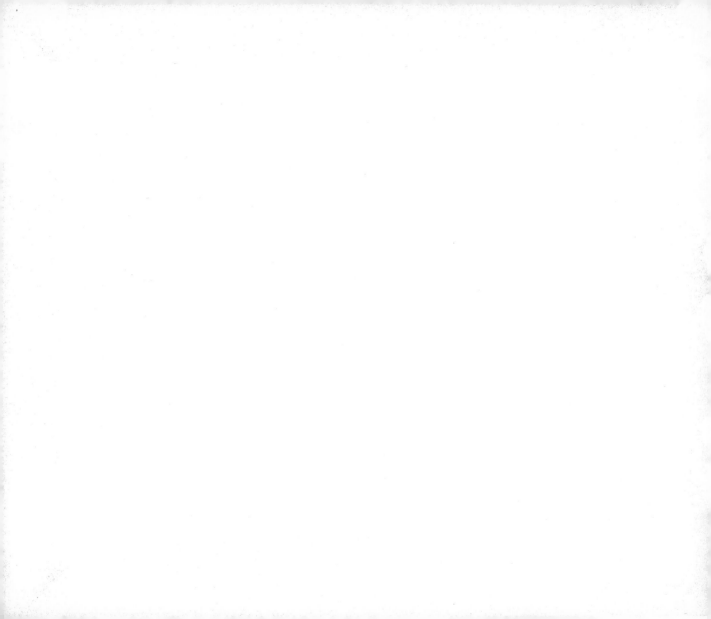

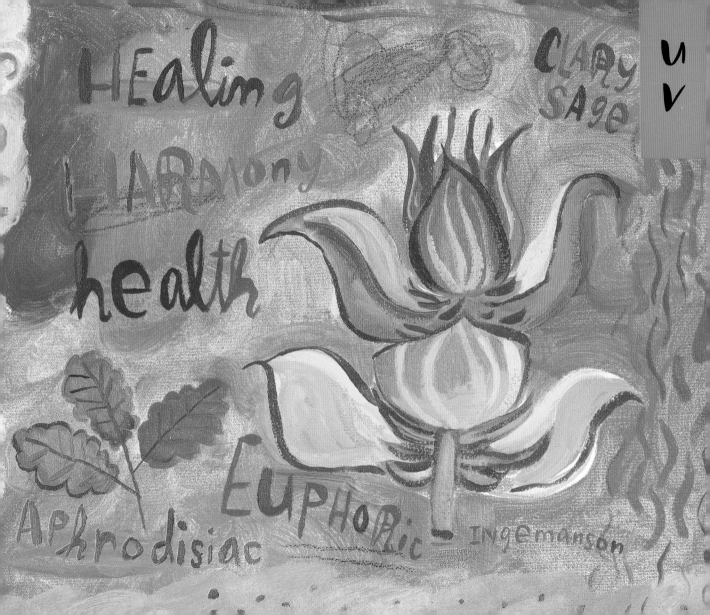

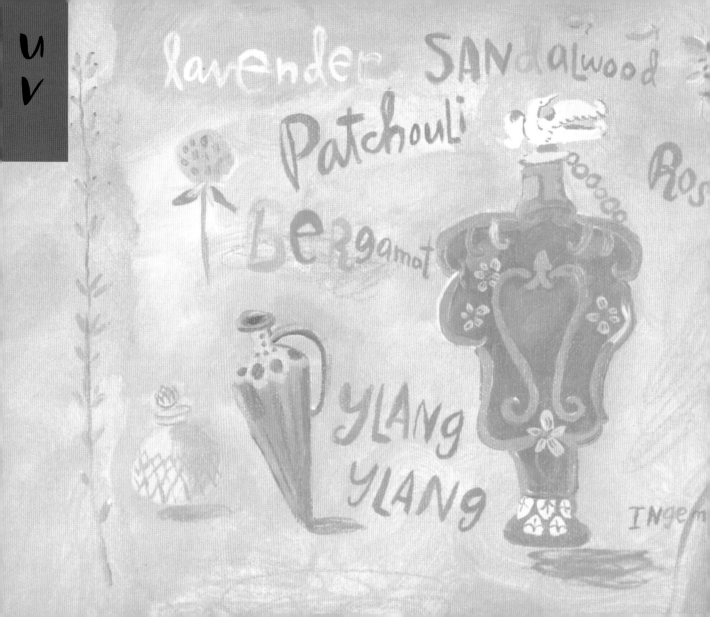

ULCERS

Bergamot, chamomile, frankincense*, geranium, lemon, myrrh (mouth), orange (mouth), rose

GASTRIC

Geranium*

STOMACH

Bergamot, frankincense, geranium, orange, peppermint. Use as food flavoring; apply to stomach.

ULCERATIONS (CLEANSE LIVER AND COLON)

Lavender, rose

VARICOSE ULCERS (SEE VARICOSE ULCERS)

UPLIFTING

Bergamot, birch, fir (emotionally uplifting), grapefruit, helichrysum, jasmine, lavender, myrrh, orange, spruce, and wild tansy
Blend: Combine 3 drops birch, 3 drops lavender, 3 drops orange, 3 drops spruce, and 1 oz. pure vegetable oil.

URETER

INFECTION

Lemon*, myrtle*

URINARY TRACT

Lavender, melaleuca, sage*, sandalwood*, rosemary, tarragon, thyme* (infection)

GENERAL

Bergamot*, eucalyptus* (general stimulant)

INFECTION

Cedarwood*, tarragon

STONES

Fennel*, geranium*

UTERUS

Cedarwood, geranium, jasmine, lemon, myrrh

UTEROTONIC

Thyme

UTERINE CANCER *(SEE CANCER)*
>Frankincense, geranium
>Blend #1: Combine 2 to 5 drops Cedarwood in 1 tsp. pure vegetable oil.
>Blend #2: Combine 2 to 5 drops lemon in 1 tsp. pure vegetable oil.
>Blend #3: Combine 2 to 5 drops myrrh in 1 tsp. pure vegetable oil.

VAGINAL

CANDIDA (THRUSH)
>Bergamot*, melaleuca*, myrrh*

INFECTION
>Cinnamon, clary sage, cypress, eucalyptus, hyssop, juniper, lavender, rosemary, sage, thyme

INFLAMMATION OF VAGINA
>Eucalyptus, lavender, melaleuca

VAGINITIS
>Cinnamon* (be careful), eucalyptus, oregano, rosemary*, rosewood*, thyme; may use a few drops in douche; apply to lower abdomen and lower back.

VARICOSE ULCERS

>Eucalyptus, geranium, lavender, melaleuca, thyme

VARICOSE VEINS

>Bergamot, cypress, helichrysum, juniper, lavender, lemon*, lemongrass*, peppermint. Helichrysum dissolves the coagulated blood inside and outside of the veins. Cypress strengthens the veins. Massage varicose veins toward the heart with helichrysum and cypress every morning and night; wear support hose until healed. It takes 2 to 3 months to heal completely.

VASCULAR SYSTEM

(ALL THE VEINS)
>Cypress, frankincense, helichrysum, lemongrass* (strengthens vascular walls); apply as a full-body massage to heart and bottoms of feet.

VEINS

CIRCULATION IN VASCULAR WALLS

Lemon

VERTIGO

(SEE EARS, EQUILIBRIUM, AND DIZZINESS)

Ginger

VIRAL DISEASE

Cinnamon bark

ANTIVIRAL

Oregano

INFECTION

Melaleuca, oregano, ravensara, thyme;
apply along spine, bottoms of feet, diffuse.

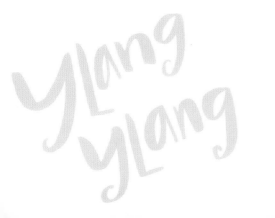

VIRUSES

Massage oregano along the spine. Also use
bergamot, cypress, eucalyptus, lavender,
melaleuca (viral and fungal infection),
ravensara (viral infection), rosemary*. Do
raindrop therapy.

ASTHMA *(SEE ASTHMA)*

EBOLA VIRUS

This virus cannot live in the presence of
cinnamon or oregano.

RESPIRATORY

Eucalyptus

SPINE

Mix 5 drops oregano and 5 drops thyme.
Put on bottoms of feet and apply raindrop
therapy on the spine.

VISUALIZATION

Helichrysum

VITAL CENTERS

Oregano and sage may strengthen the vital
centers of the body.

VOICE (HOARSE)

Jasmine

VOMITING

(SEE NAUSEA)

Fennel*, nutmeg, peppermint (aromatic)
Massage or compress over stomach:
Chamomile, fennel, lavender, pepper
(black), peppermint, rose

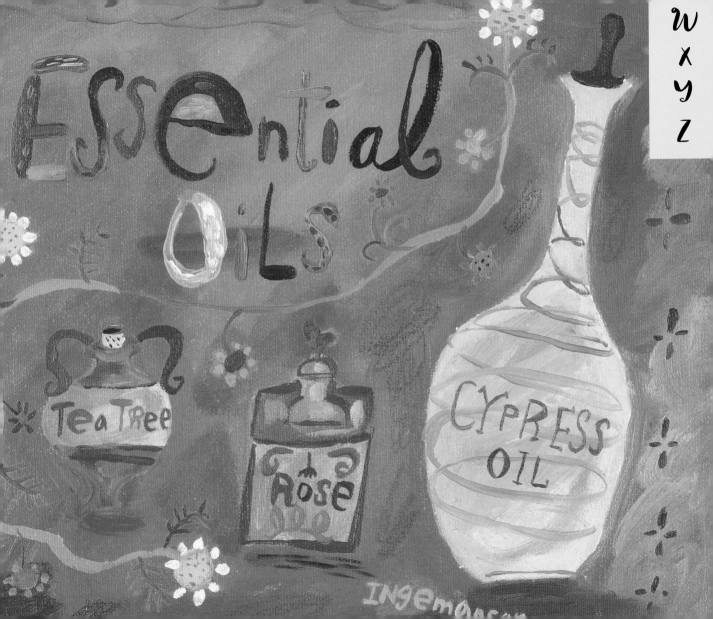

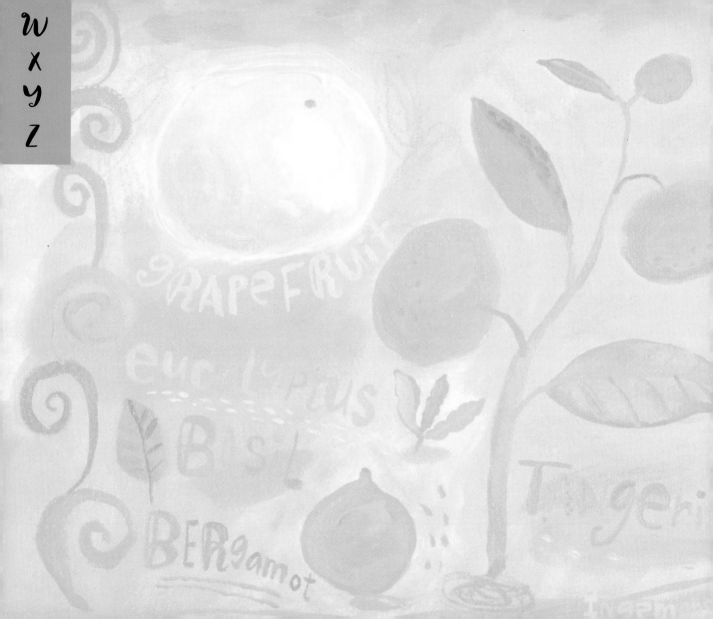

WXYZ

GRAPEFRUIT

eucalyptus

Basil

Bergamot

Tangeri

WARTS

Cinnamon, cypress, frankincense, jasmine, lavender, lemon (may dilute in 2 tsps. cider vinegar), oregano
Blend: Combine 5 drops cypress, 10 drops lemon, 2 Tbls. apple cider vinegar, A, D & E tincture. Apply twice daily and bandage; keep a bandage on it until wart is gone.

PLANTAR
Oregano

WASTE

ELIMINATING
Lavender (through lymphatic system)

WATER DISTILLATION

Add 3 to 5 drops of your favorite oil to the postfilter on your distiller. The oils will help increase the oxygen and frequency of the water. Try birch, cinnamon, lemon, and peppermint.

WATER PURIFICATION

Lemon*, orange

REMOVE NITRATES
Peppermint

WATER RETENTION
(SEE EDEMA AND HORMONAL IMBALANCE)

WEAKNESS

AFTER ILLNESS
Thyme (physical)

WEALTH

Bergamot

ATTRACTS
Cinnamon bark (aromatic)

MONEY
Ginger, patchouly

WEIGHT
(SEE HORMONAL IMBALANCE)

OVERWEIGHT

The following may contribute to the problem of overweight: slow metabolism, lack of exercise, low fiber, poor diet, stress, enzyme deficiency, hormonal imbalance, low thyroid function, and poor digestion and assimilation.

Blend #1: Put 5 drops lemon and grapefruit in 1 gallon of water and drink during the day. Add more grapefruit to dissolve fat faster.

Blend #2: Combine 4 drops lavender, 4 drops basil, 3 drops juniper, 8 drops grapefruit, 5 drops cypress; mix and apply to feet, on location, as a body massage, or use in bath. Blend is used to emulsify fat.

Tea: Lapacho tea made with distilled water; drink lots of water.

WELL-BEING
Rose, wild tansy

FEELING OF

Spearmint

PROMOTES

Eucalyptus, lemon

WHOOPING COUGH
(SEE CHILDHOOD DISEASES)

Cinnamon, clary sage, cypress, grapefruit, hyssop, lavender, oregano*; apply on chest, throat.

Diffuse: Basil, chamomile, eucalyptus, lavender, melaleuca, peppermint, rose, thyme

WITHDRAWAL
(SEE ADDICTIONS)

WORKAHOLIC
Basil, geranium, lavender, marjoram

WORMS

Bergamot, chamomile, lavender, melaleuca, melissa, peppermint, thyme
Blend: Mix 6 drops chamomile (Roman), 6 drops eucalyptus, 6 drops lavender, and 6 drops lemon with 2 Tbls. pure vegetable oil.

WORRY

Bergamot

WOUNDS

Bergamot, chamomile, clove* (infected wounds), eucalyptus, frankincense, juniper, lavender, myrrh, rose, rosemary, rosewood, thyme

WEEPING

Juniper, patchouly, tarragon
Blend: Combine 5 drops chamomile, 10 drops lavender, 3 drops tarragon, and 2 oz. pure vegetable oil; hot compress.

HEALING

Melaleuca (pus-filled wounds), ravensara

WRINKLES

Clary sage, fennel, frankincense, geranium, lavender, lemon, myrrh, orange, oregano, patchouly, rose, rosemary, sandalwood, thyme
Blend #1: Combine 3 drops lavender, 4 drops geranium, 2 drops patchouly, 6 drops rosewood, and 1 oz. pure vegetable oil. Rub on wrinkles.
Blend #2: Mix 1 drop frankincense, 1 drop lavender, and 1 drop lemon. It's like magic for wrinkles. Rub on morning and night around eyes.

YEAST
(SEE CANDIDA)

YOGA

Sandalwood

ZEST (FOR LIFE)

Nutmeg (aromatic)

Bibliography

Balch, James, and Phyllis Balch. *Prescription for Nutritional Healing*. Garden City Park, NY: Avery Publishing Group, 1990.

Burroughs, Stanley. *Healing for the Age of Enlightenment*. Auburn, CA: Burroughs Books, 1993.

Burton Goldberg Group, The. *Alternative Medicine: The Definitive Guide*. Fife, WA: Future Medicine Publishing, Inc., 1994.

Dodt, Colleen K. *The Essential Oil Book: Creating Personal Blends for Mind & Body*. Pownal, VT: Storey Communications, Inc., 1996.

Fischer-Rizzi, Suzanne. *Complete Aromatherapy Handbook*. New York: Sterling Publishing, 1990.

Friedmann, Terry Spencer. *Freedom Through Health*. Scottsdale, AZ: Harvest Publishing, 1993.

Lawless, Julia. *The Encyclopaedia of Essential Oils*. Rockport, MA: Element, Inc., 1992.

Rose, Jeanne. *The Aromatherapy Book: Applications and Inhalations*. Berkeley, CA: North Atlantic Books, 1992.

Selby, Anna. *Aromatherapy*. New York, NY: Macmillan, 1996.

Tisserand, Maggie. *Aromatherapy for Women: A Practical Guide to Essential Oils for Health and Beauty*. Rochester, VT: Healing Arts Press, 1996.

Tisserand, Robert. *Aromatherapy: To Heal and Tend the Body*. Wilmot, WI: Lotus Press, 1988.

Tisserand, Robert. *The Art of Aromatherapy*. Rochester, VT: Healing Arts Press, 1977.

Valnet, Jean. *The Practice of Aromatherapy: A Classic Compendium of Plant Medicines and their Healing Properties*. Rochester, VT: Healing Arts Press, 1980.

Wilson, Roberta. *Aromatherapy for Vibrant Health and Beauty: A practical A-to-Z reference to aromatherapy treatments for health, skin, and hair problems*. Honesdale, PA: Paragon Press, 1995.

Worwood, Valerie Ann. *The Complete Book of Essential Oils & Aromatherapy*. San Rafael, CA: New World Library, 1991.

Young, D. Gary. *Aromatherapy: The Essential Beginning*. Salt Lake City, UT: Essential Press Publishing, 1995.

About the Authors

PAT LEATHAM has been searching for natural healing methods all her life. From her birth until she was about 14 years old, she was constantly sick, finding just a little relief from her illnesses during her high school years. She suffered annual appendicitis attacks for 12 years and was always told by the medical profession that they couldn't operate because she was too sick. Because of these experiences and several others, she developed a fascination for natural healing methods. Her search really began at about the age of 14 when she would comb through her brother's Boy Scout magazines for wild plants that were beneficial for various things. She even compiled these notes into a book of her own. From there, her search expanded. In 1961, she completed her two-year certification on the Principles of Personology. After raising a family of six children, she received certifications in Rapid Eye Technology in 1992 and In-Depth Educational Kinesiology in 1993. Still propelled by her fascination for natural healing methods, she started her study of aromatherapy in January 1995. In May of that same year, she met Connie and shared the notes she had taken at lectures and conferences, from videos and audiotapes, and from many discussions with others. She then solicited Connie's help in organizing and expanding that information.

CONNIE HIGLEY has also had a fascination for natural healing methods, relying on herbs and herbal remedies for much of her life. Always interested in natural ways to help maintain the health of her family, she has studied Educational Kinesiology and attended several lectures and conferences on natural healing methods. Having a unique talent for organizing information, she received her bachelor's degree in Information Management in 1989. As a devoted mother, Connie became excited about the possible uses of essential oils when she learned about the therapeutic and emotional effects that could be achieved by topical application and inhalation rather than ingestion. In May 1995, she met Pat Leatham and was shown the pages of notes that Pat had compiled over the previous four months. Connie worked with Pat to organize the information, and then she expanded it for the two of them and their friends. The growing demand for this information has evolved into this book and others. Because of Connie's tremendous desire to help others by providing needed, well-organized information, she summoned the help of her husband, Alan, and together they continue to research and expand this vital information.

We hope you enjoyed this Hay House Lifestyles book.

If you would like to receive a free catalog featuring additional Hay House books and products, or if you would like information about the Hay Foundation, please contact:

Hay House, Inc.
P.O. Box 5100
Carlsbad, CA 92018-5100
(760) 431-7695 or (800) 654-5126
(760) 431-6948 (fax) or (800) 650-5115 (fax)

Please visit the Hay House Website at:
www.hayhouse.com

Hay House Australia Pty Ltd.
P.O. Box 515
Brighton-Le-Sands, NSW 2216
phone: 1800 023 516
e-mail: info@hayhouse.com.au

M8072-C
66   TN